Social Work with Lesbian I

The traditional concept of family as being exclusively heterosexual has resulted in myth-generation about lesbian parents as well as fostering limitations in the programs and benefits that support more diverse nontraditional families. *Social Work with Lesbian Parent Families: Ecological Perspectives* explores the variety of social systems with which lesbian parent families interact, with a focus on implications for improved, diversity-affirming service delivery and policy development. Unlike other literature on lesbian parent families, this revealing resource pulls together work on lesbian parenting from various researchers across a broad range of disciplines and presents this work from the ecosystems perspective so that the reader may view the experiences of lesbian parent families in a holistic way.

The research goes beyond simple comparisons between lesbian and straight mothers. This useful text provides more complex research data, including both a more sophisticated view of the diverse communities in which lesbian parents are found, and more innovative ways of studying the issues relevant to social service providers. Developmental and life issues negotiated by lesbian parent families are discussed in detail using a strengths-based approach to intervention with individuals, families, small groups, communities, and larger systems. This unique book has the strong potential to influence the policies that impact lesbian parent families.

Social Work with Lesbian Parent Families: Ecological Perspectives is a valuable resource for social workers, psychologists, sociologists, anthropologists, marriage and family therapists, public policy and administration professionals, students, and academics doing research on sexual orientation and family.

This book was published as a special issue of the *Journal of Gay & Lesbian Social Services*.

Lucy R. Mercier is Associate Professor of Social Work and Youth Services and Field Education Coordinator at Saginaw Valley State University.

Rena D. Harold is Professor and Associate Director of the School of Social Work at Michigan State University.

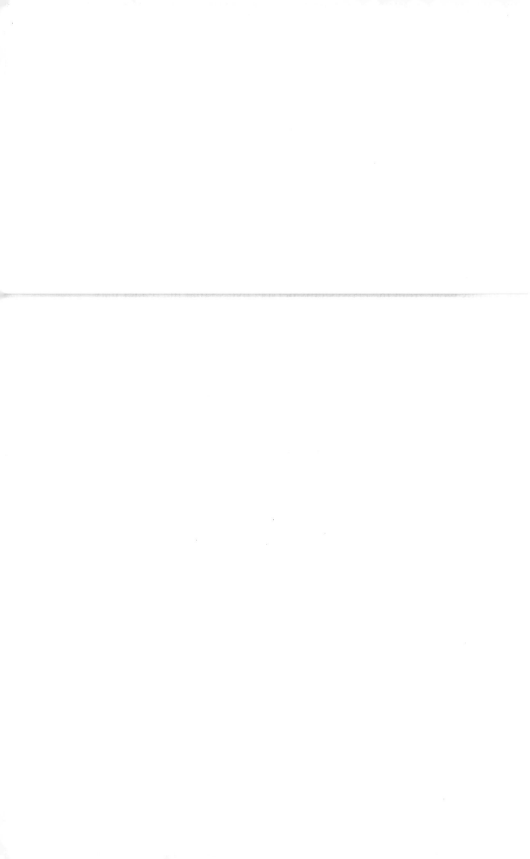

Social Work with Lesbian Parent Families

Ecological Perspectives

Edited by Lucy R. Mercier and Rena D. Harold

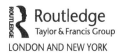
Routledge
Taylor & Francis Group

LONDON AND NEW YORK

First published 2009 by Routledge
2 Park Square, Milton Park, Abingdon, Oxfordshire OX14 4RN

Simultaneously published in the USA and Canada
by Routledge
711 Third Avenue, New York, NY 10017

First issued in paperback 2015

Routledge is an imprint of the Taylor & Francis Group, an informa business

Typeset in Times by Value Chain, India

British Library Cataloguing in Publication Data
A catalogue record for this book is available from the British Library

ISBN 13: 978-1-138-86757-4 (pbk)
ISBN 13: 978-1-5602-3755-6 (hbk)

CONTENTS

> *Ninety-six lesbian adoptive parents were part of a cross-sectional study to explore their adoption experiences, specifically focusing on their sources of consultation/information and possible bias, adoption timeframes and costs, and their satisfaction with the adoption experience. Questions within each of these domains were tested for significant differences across international, private domestic and child welfare adoption venues. While their overall experiences were positive, several key significant findings are discussed, with practice considerations suggested for adoption professionals and other lesbians seeking adoption. Lastly, a call for future research is made to further our understanding of lesbian mothers' transition to adoptive parenthood.*

> *Twenty-one lesbian parents, representing 15 families, were interviewed to examine the work-family issues experienced by the women. Seventy percent of the interviewees were satisfied with their employment situations and characterized the relationships between their households and the workplace as positive. Qualitative analysis of the interview data revealed work-related stressors and supports, and strategies for balancing work and family. Themes included instrumental support, interpersonal support, integration of work and family, and creative responses to work-family tensions. Implications for social work policy and direct practice are discussed.*

> *Judicial decisions, especially Supreme Court decisions, are becoming, more than ever, major contributors to social policy creation. The political implications*

of such decisions have far reaching implications for policy analysts, advocates, systems, and individuals. *In the case of* Goodridge v. Department of Public Health (*2003*), *the state asked the court to limit the civil rights of a certain group of people because of their sexual orientation. Despite the impact court decisions have on policy, there are few models designed to be used to connect the impact of court decisions to the societal and personal values that underlie them. This paper describes a new model designed by the author to analyze judicial decisions, one that includes a value critical approach, and shows its application to the* Goodridge (*2003*) *ruling granting same sex couples the right to legally marry in Massachusetts.*

This article discusses the impact of lesbian mothers' activism on legislation and personal well-being. Using a meaning reconstruction framework, the activism of lesbian parents is evaluated as a source of resilience and strength in the current political climate. A case history of one community where lesbian mothers formed a local coalition in response to a statewide proposition to ban same-sex marriage in Texas is described. This community example shows how the activism of lesbian parents can transform both community and activists. Implications for community organizers, therapists and LGBT parents/allies are discussed.

Barriers to services for lesbians and their families have been well documented in the literature (DeCrescenzo, 1984; Harris, Schatz, & O'Hanlan, 1994; Nightengale, & Owen, 1995; Mallon, 1998), especially among medical professionals and social service providers. This study seeks to explore the prevalence of heterosexism and homophobia among mental health practitioners who identify as qualified providers for lesbians and the recipients' perspectives regarding the services they have received. Of the twenty-five practitioners who responded, 48% of them "knew personally of incidences of professional bias against lesbian clients." Interestingly, only 26% of the 98 families reported heterosexual bias from their providers.

About the Contributors

Sandra C. Anderson, PhD, is Professor in the Graduate School of Social Work at Portland State University. She has had a private practice for over 20 years in which she works with many lesbians and their families.

Mindy Holliday, MA, MSW, is Assistant Professor in the Graduate School of Social Work at Portland State University. Her research focus is on gay/lesbian issues, multicultural practice, and ethnographic research on women's lives.

Barbara L. Jones, PhD, MSW, is Assistant Professor at the UT Austin School of Social Work where she is also Co-Director of The Institute for Grief, Loss and Family Survival. Dr. Jones was the Principal Investigator on a study entitled, *Voices of Struggle: Understanding and Memorializing the Fight Against Constitutional Amendment #2* and is currently a member of the Council on Sexual Orientation and Gender Expression at the Council of Social Work Education. Dr. Jones is a Project on Death in America Social Work Scholar and conducts research on issues related to grief, loss, and resilience.

Lucy R. Mercier, PhD, is Associate Professor of Social Work and Youth Services and Field Education Coordinator at Saginaw Valley State University. She is a member of the Council on the Role and Status of Women at the Council of Social Work Education. Her research focuses on family development and lesbian parent family systems. A licensed social worker, her community involvement includes work with GLBT family support and advocacy organizations.

Scott Ryan, PhD, is Associate Professor and Associate Dean at Florida State University's College of Social Work, and is also Director of the Institute for Social Work Research. In addition, he is a Senior Research Fellow with the Evan B. Donaldson Adoption Institute. Lastly, he is the Editor of the journal, *Adoption Quarterly*. Through his work, Dr. Ryan has led several high-impact research projects on a wide array of adoption-related topics, including adoptee identity development, children's development in adoptive families headed by same-sex parents, and post-adoption support services.

Tanya M. Voss, LCSW, is Clinical Assistant Professor and Director of Field Education at the University of Texas at Austin School of Social Work. Ms. Voss was one of the key researchers on the *Voices of Struggle* study and she works with disenfranchised and complicated grief in her groups for children of incarcerated parents in juvenile justice-based settings. In 2003, Ms. Voss was a recipient of the Family Pride Coalition's Family of Courage Award, created to honor those who have taken on the challenges presented by unfriendly courts and/or legislatures and worked to create a better, safer place for LGBT parents and their children.

Misty L. Wall, MSSW, LCSW, PhD Candidate, is concluding her doctoral research at the University of Texas at Arlington School of Social Work. She also provides individual, group, and family therapy through the Women's Center of Tarrant County and is an adjunct professor at University of Texas at Arlington.

Courtney Whitlock received a Bachelor's in Social Work from Florida State University in 2006. Currently, she is a student at Hofstra University's School of Law where she received a fellowship in Family and Child Advocacy.

Preface:
We *Are* Family:
Lesbian Parenting

Research into lesbian parenting has moved well beyond the earliest studies, when comparisons between lesbian and straight mothers were common. As this field has matured, research questions have become more complex, often including both a more sophisticated view of the diverse communities in which lesbian parents are found and more innovative ways of studying the issues relevant to social service providers. This volume explores and describes a variety of social systems with which lesbian parent families interact, with a focus on implications for improved, diversity-affirming service delivery and policy.

The most commonly cited statistics concerning the number of gay and lesbian parents in the United States range from two to eight million (Patterson, 1995b), but accurate estimates of the actual numbers of lesbian mothers are difficult to find. Some researchers estimate that there are between 6 million and 14 million children with at least one gay or lesbian parent (Johnson & O'Conner, 2002). Despite gains in broadening the definition of family, these parents still struggle under a conception of family that is primarily heterosexual. And as increasing numbers of lesbians choose motherhood (Johnson & O'Conner, 2002), it is important to understand the experiences of these women and their families. As single and coupled lesbians are choosing to participate in this adult developmental life transition, many legal scholars and children's advocacy organizations have advocated for a societal redefinition of the family in such a way that lesbians would be included within the legal definition (Cianciotto & Cahill, 2003). However, many continue to believe that "as long as family–in whatever form it takes–remains a dominant legal category, lesbians are positioned as either outlaws or in-laws" (Robson, 1994, p. 993).

What fuels the latter argument is the notion that it is necessary to change more than a definition if real social change is to take place. The concept of family as heterosexual is a product of laws that are based on religious values and beliefs (Poverney & Finch, 1988). The law controls access to marriage, thus imposing traditional definitions of the family. In turn, these definitions shape the infrastructure of programs and the benefits that support families. In addition, lesbian parents have had to deal with common myths held by many in society, e.g., lesbians are less maternal than their heterosexual counterparts and therefore are poorer mothers (Lewin, 1993). Despite the fact that these myths have been dispelled by research (e.g., Flaks, Ficher, Masterpasqua, & Joseph, 1995; Kirkpatrick, 1987; Laird, 1993; Patterson, 1995a), lesbians continue to have to defend themselves against these ideas.

In 1988, Poverney and Finch wrote, "most futurists agree that the family, as a social construct, is expanding to include more diverse forms" (p. 116). As definitions of family have moved away from conventional constraints in structure and function, new knowledge has emerged that emphasizes an understanding of family as a complex and changeable arena for the working through and development of interpersonal, economic, political, and other relations (Ferree, 1991; Laird, 1993; Lewin, 1993; Robson, 1994).

In addition to documenting the experiences of these women and their families in an attempt to create a "picture" of them and to explore what issues they identify as important in the development of their family, it is also important to focus on the social policy implications of and for lesbian parenting in this volume. Misty Wall's article, "A Model for Policy Analysis Applied to the Goodridge Case," demonstrates one paradigm for exploring the impact of public policy on lesbian parents and their families. The article by Scott Ryan and Courtney Whitlock,' "Becoming Parents: Lesbian Mothers' Adoption Experience," discusses how these families experience agency policy and practice in the arena of adoption.

Some studies have explored the unique structures and processes of lesbian mother families without focusing on comparison with other groups. Early work in this area included material on adoption, donor insemination and foster parenting, legal issues for lesbian mothers, co-parenting, and family-of-origin reactions to lesbian mother families

(Pies, 1988). Subsequently, the literature has outlined areas of potential difficulty for lesbian mothers including the role of employment and money in parenting decisions, the impact of children on adult intimacy, and the role of gender in lesbians' decisions to parent (Martin 1993; Pies, 1988). Lucy Mercier's article, "Lesbian Parents and Work: Stressors and Supports for the Work-Family Interface," focuses on employment benefits and the relationships between parenting and work decisions.

Lesbian mother families are impacted by the lesbian community as well as by mainstream culture and expectations. Some portions of the lesbian community are experienced as "anti-family, anti-children" (Lott-Whitehead & Tully, 1993, p. 276), but other studies have shown that friendship networks and community support provided the majority of support for these families (Ainslie & Feltey, 1991; Weston, 1991). Barbara Jones and Tanya Voss consider some of these issues in their article, "Lesbian Parent Activism and Meaning-Making in the Current Political Environment: One Community's Story."

Clinical social workers and other service providers continue to struggle in their relationships with lesbian parent families, as evidenced by literature that often exhorts professionals to confront individual and institutional heterosexism and to increase education about lesbian mothers' special needs and resources (Berkman & Zinberg, 1997; Dahlheimer & Feigal, 1991; Erlichman, 1988; Kirkpatrick, 1987). A few writers have addressed clinical issues relevant to lesbian mother families more specifically, including the emerging importance of family ritual in gay and lesbian families (Markowitz, 1991), competition over providing and receiving nurturing, acceptance by extended family, and lesbian family dissolution (Chambers, 1998; Morton, 1998). Sandra Anderson and Mindy Holliday's article, "How Heterosexism Plagues Practitioners in Services for Lesbians and Their Families: An Exploratory Study," addresses some of the continuing questions regarding the role of professional helpers in working with lesbian-led families.

While important research on mainstream families continues, a more thorough understanding of alternative families is vital to the continuing development of knowledge in social work and the other helping professions. In particular, the study of families that vary by the sexual orientation of their members is important because of its relationship to issues as diverse as gender roles in family life, understanding of family composition and purpose, the impact of social support and social policy on family life, and the role of individual experience in the success of families. Lesbian-mother families "provide a fertile testing ground for family theories and simultaneously pose . . . challenges for dominant family theories" (Demo & Allen, 1996. p. 423). Teaching about contemporary families is enhanced by a conceptual model that embraces lesbian-mother families as innovators in the changing climate of the academy, family politics, and social structures. Lesbian mother families constitute a significant population, and the use of data on lesbian mother families in the classroom supports learning about sexual and racial-ethnic diversity, family structure, class, gender, and power.

This volume pulls together work on lesbian parent families from various researchers to present this collection from the ecosystems perspective, so that the reader may view the experiences of lesbian parent families in a holistic way. This broader perspective on the developmental and life issues negotiated by lesbian parent families lends itself naturally to a strengths-based approach to intervention with individuals, families, small groups, communities, and larger systems. In addition, it has the potential to influence social policy that affects lesbian parent families and other non-traditional family forms.

Lucy R. Mercier
Rena D. Harold

REFERENCES

Ainslie, J. & Feltey, K. M. (1991). Definition and dynamics of motherhood and family in lesbian communities. *Marriage and Family Review, 17* (1-2), 63-85.

Berkman, C. & Zinberg, G. (1997). Homophobia and heterosexism in social workers. *Social Work, 42* (4), 319-332.

Chambers, D. L. (1998). Lesbian divorce: A commentary on legal issues. *American Journal of Orthopsychiatry, 68* (3), 420-423.

Cianciotto, J, & Cahill, S. (2003). *Education policy: Issues affecting lesbian, gay, bisexual and transgender youth.* New York: The National Gay and Lesbian Task Force Policy Institute. Available at: http://www.thetaskforce.org/downloads/EducationPolicy.pdf

Dahlheimer, D. & Feigal, J. (1991). Bridging the gap. *Family Therapy Networker, 15* (1), 44-53.

Demo, D. and Allen, K. (1996). Diversity within lesbian and gay families: Challenges and implications for family theory and research. *Journal of Social and Personal Relations, 13* (3), 415-434.

Erlichman, K. (1988). Lesbian mothers: Ethical issues in social work practice. *Women and Therapy, 8,* 207-224.

Ferree, M. (1991). Beyond separate spheres: Feminism and family research. In A. Booth (Ed.), *Contemporary families: Looking forward, looking back.* (pp. 103-121). Minneapolis: National Council on Family Relations.

Flaks, D. K., Ficher, I., Masterpasqua, F., & Joseph, G. (1995). Lesbians choosing motherhood: A comparative study of lesbian and heterosexual parents and their children. *Developmental Psychology, 31*, 105-114.

Johnson, S. M., & O'Conner, E. (2002). *The gay baby boom.* New York: New York University Press.

Kirkpatrick, M. (1987). Clinical implications of lesbian mother studies. *Journal of Homosexuality, 14*, 201-211.

Laird, J. (1993). Lesbian and gay families. In F. Walsh (Ed.), *Normal family processess, 2nd Edition.* (pp 176-210). New York: Guilford.

Lewin, E. (1993). *Lesbian mothers: Accounts of gender in American culture.* Ithaca, NY: Cornell University Press.

Lott-Whitehead, L., & Tully, C. (1993). The family lives of lesbian mothers. *Smith College Studies in Social Work, 63* (3), 265-280.

Markowitz, L. (1991). Homosexuality: Are we still in the dark? *Networker, 15* (1), 26-35.

Martin, A. (1993). *The lesbian and gay parenting handbook: Creating and raising our families.* New York: HarperCollins.

Morton, S. B. (1998). Lesbian divorce. *American Journal of Orthopsychiatry, 68* (3), 410-419.

Patterson, C. J. (1995a). *Lesbian and gay parenting: A resource for psychologists.* Washington: American Psychological Association. Available at http://www.apa.org/pi/parent.html

Patterson, C. J. (1995b). Lesbian mothers, gay fathers and their children. In A. R. D'Augelli & C. J. Patterson (Eds.), *Lesbian, gay and bisexual identities over the lifespan.* New York: Oxford Press.

Pies, C. (1988). *Considering parenthood* (2nd ed.). Minneapolis, MN: Spinsters Ink.

Poverney, L. M., & Finch, W. A. (1988). Gay and lesbian domestic partnerships: Expanding the definition of family. *Social Casework, 69*, 116-121.

Robson, R. (1994). Resisting the family: Repositioning lesbians in legal theory. *Signs, 19*, 975-996.

Weston, K. (1991). *Families we choose: Lesbians, gays and kinship.* New York: Columbia University Press.

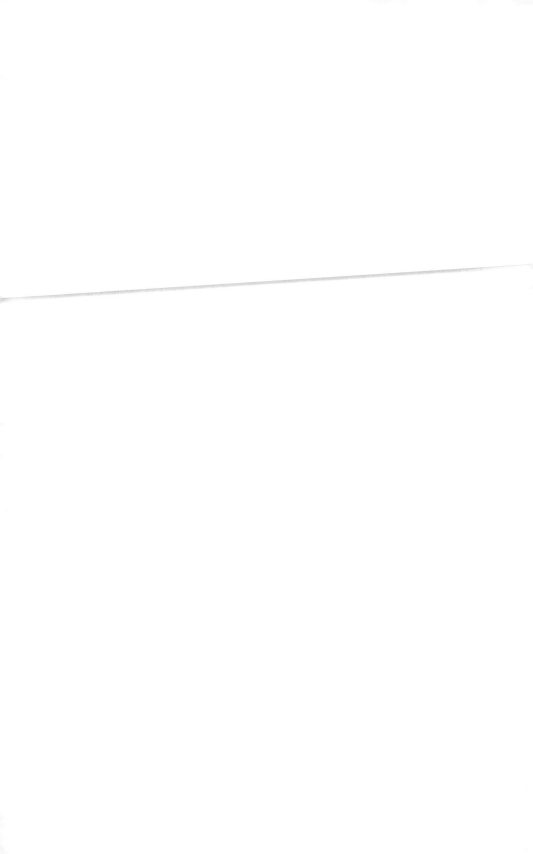

Becoming Parents:
Lesbian Mothers' Adoption Experience

Scott Ryan
Courtney Whitlock

INTRODUCTION

Adoption is the method provided by law that establishes the legal relationship of parent and child between persons, not typically related through birth, with the same mutual rights and obligations that exist between children and their birth parents. Families seeking to adopt a child can do so though one of three paths: international adoptions, public child welfare adoptions, or domestic private adoptions.

The popularity of international adoptions has steadily increased over the years, with approximately 22,000 immigration visas issued for foreign orphans adopted by families in the United States in 2005 (Time, 2006). In addition to those children adopted internationally, in 2003, the most recent year data are available, over 120,000 children were awaiting adoption in the public child welfare system. The number of children in foster care available for adoption has hovered around this amount since 2000, despite almost 50,000 children adopted annually within that same time period (Child Welfare League of America, 2006).

While data on the number of international and child welfare adoptions are available, data from private agencies are currently not being systematically collected. According to Elizabeth Betts, Child Welfare Information Associate at the National Adoption Information Clearinghouse, there is no single source for the total number of children adopted in the United States, and currently there is no straightforward way of determining the total number of such adoptions, even when multiple sources of data are used as no one agency is charged with compiling information on all private adoptions in the United States (Elizabeth Betts, personal communication, March 6, 2006). Nevertheless, as reported by Kreider (2003), approximately 2.5% of all children in the United States are adopted from one source or another. As such, it is clear that the adoption of children from all three sources comprises a significant amount of the population.

As the number of completed adoptions as well as the continuing need for adoptive families has increased, the constellation of families seeking to adopt children has become more diverse, with adoptive family structures diverging from the traditional two-parent heterosexual adoptive family. In the year 2003, the most recent data available, married families comprised only 61% of families adopting children from the child welfare system (CWLA, 2006). Twenty-six percent were single women, single men adopted 3% of the time, and unmarried couples accounted for 1% of adoptions, with data pertaining to the remaining 9% unavailable (CWLA, 2006). Similar findings were reported for adoptions using data collected via the census, with 78% of adoptive families comprised of married households, 5% percent unmarried male-headed households, and 17% unmarried female-headed households (Kreider, 2003).

While the time spent by children waiting for an adoptive placement has steadily increased (CWLA, 2006), applicants previously overlooked and/or barred, such as lesbian women, the population of interest for this study, have begun adopting children. Black, Gates, Sanders and Taylor (2000) estimate that 2.5% of the population is comprised of gay men and 1.4% of lesbian women. Given these data, it is reasonable to assume that gay men and lesbians adopt at least several hundred children annually (Ryan, in press) although even this estimation is thought to be low, as many gay or lesbian persons in committed relationships may adopted singly and thus be underrepresented. Nevertheless, numerous barriers to such adoptions persist (Ryan, Pearlmutter & Groza, 2004). Currently, Florida is the only state that explicitly bans gay and lesbians from adopting children (Appell, 2003). However, other states have also erected barriers. In Utah, for example, persons who are cohabiting, but not legally married, may not adopt. This indirectly excludes gay and lesbian persons due to the fact that the law does not recognize their unions. As this issue has become a matter of public attention and interest, one survey questioned Floridian's opinion of this ban with the findings indicating that 67% of the respondents (n = 413) support gay and lesbian persons being considered as an adoption resource (Ryan, Bedard, & Gertz, 2004).

Based on the research evidence available, as well as the recognition of the great need for homes for the thousands of children awaiting an adoptive placement, many professional associations have taken clear positions regarding the inclusion of gay and lesbian adults as possible adoptive resources. At the forefront is the Child Welfare League of America, the nation's oldest and largest child advocacy group, that states in its Standards for Excellence for Adoption Services that: "Applicants should be assessed on the basis of their ability to successfully parent a child needing family membership and not on their race, ethnicity or culture, income, age, marital status, religion, appearance, differing lifestyles or sexual orientation" (CWLA, 2000, p. 50). They further assert that, "Sexual preference [sic] should not be the sole criteria on which the suitability of the adoptive applicants is based. Consideration should be given to other personality and maturity factors and on the ability of the applicant to meet the specific needs of the individual child" (p. 50). Similar positions have been taken by the National Association of Social Workers (2000), the American Psychiatric Association (1986), the American Psychological Association (1975, 1976), the American Academy of Pediatrics (2002), the American Academy of Child and Adolescent Psychiatry (1999), the American Psychoanalytic Association (2002), and the North American Council on Adoptable Children (2002).

Given the numbers of children adopted and available for adoption, this research seeks to gain more information on the adoptive experience for lesbian women. Specifically, it will attempt to examine the overall satisfaction and potential barriers these individuals encounter during the adoption process, and, when data are available, to examine whether the barriers faced are unique to this population or universal to all adoptive applicants. Lastly, these experiences will be explored across adoption type (international, child welfare, private domestic) to determine if any one form has been more open and accepting of this population.

LITERATURE REVIEW

The literature review was completed using a systematic research synthesis (SRS) of the available empirical literature on adopted children. An SRS is a critical review of the literature that enables both meta-analytic methods and traditional reviews of the literature (Rothman, Damron-Rodriquez, & Shenassa, 1994). The key word searches included: adoption, homosexual adoption, lesbian adoption, minority adoption, adoption experience, adoption satisfaction, adoption costs, child welfare adoption, private adoption and international adoption. The following online databases were searched: PsychINFO, Education Resources Information Center (ERIC), Social Services Abstracts, Sociological Abstracts, and ProQuest's Dissertation Abstracts. Initially, anecdotal findings were excluded, although as the scarcity of the empirical literature became apparent, information included in the current study also came from organizations relevant to the topic of interest including, for example, the American Psychological Association, the Child Welfare League of America, and the National Adoption Information Clearinghouse.

Sources of Consultation/Information and Possible Bias

One study examined the openness of various agencies to gay and lesbian adoptive parents by mailing questionnaires to agency program directors (Brodzinsky, Patterson & Vaziri, 2002). Note that only two states, Florida and New Hampshire, banned such adoptions by statute at the time of the Brodzinsky, Patterson and Vaziri study (in April of 1999, New Hampshire repealed its 1988 ban prohibiting lesbians and gay men from becoming adoptive and foster parents). Additionally, respondents from six other states reported these adoptions as being against the law, with no such law enacted, and 29 respondents were unaware of their state's current law. However, 63% of all respondents reported acceptance of applications from gay and lesbian individuals and/or couples. According to the responses of the participants the religious affiliation of the adoption agency greatly affected its openness to gay and lesbian applicants. Overall, the agencies participating facilitated 22,584 adoptions two years prior to the study. Approximately 371 (1.6%) were known to have been placed with gay and lesbian individuals and/or couples although the respondents themselves estimated a higher rate of 2.9% due to under-reporting. While the exact number of these adoptions is unknown, the study reflects an overall attitude of acceptance and openness towards lesbian adoptive applicants.

Currently, there have been two studies assessing the opinions of child welfare workers and their impact on placement recommendations (Ryan, 2000; Taylor, 1998). Social workers' attitudes towards gay and lesbian adoptive parents were examined, with findings indicating that attitudes were a result of childhood experiences and professional training (Ryan, 2000). Taylor (1998) reported that a sample of 50 child welfare workers, overall, favored allowing adoptions by gay and lesbians. However, the sample's mean score fell into the Index of Attitudes toward Homosexuals low-grade homophobic range. Approximately one-third of respondents stated that gay and lesbian adoption applicants should not be able to adopt a child under the age of 5, and 25% held this position until the child was 15 (Taylor, 1998). It should be noted that the sampling methods of these studies severely limit the generalizability of their findings.

In a study of lesbian adoptive parents (n = 18), heterosexual adoptive parents (n = 44), and lesbian parents using in-vitro fertilization (n = 49), Shelley-Sireci and Ciano-Boyce (2002) found that the level of difficulty with the adoption process was relatively equivalent across groups. A scale using 1 as very easy, 2 somewhat easy, 3 neutral, 4 somewhat difficult, and 5 as very difficult measured this factor. Both the lesbian and heterosexual couples rated their experience as "neutral." Their overall experiences with the adoption process were also equivalent; however, the lesbian adoptive parents did perceive significantly more discrimination throughout the adoptive process as a result of their sexual orientation. When asked, *"Did you or your partner feel like you had to omit information in the homestudy in order to have a successful outcome?"* an overwhelming 81% of the lesbian mothers responded affirmatively versus the 24% of heterosexual couples.

Bausch and Serpe (1999) identified perceived obstacles to adoption with Mexican American respondents. Of the 591 Mexican American respondents, 38% indicated a likeliness to adopt, but thought that obstacles such as lack of information, resources, and bilingual social workers would make it difficult. Rodriguez and Meyer (1990) reviewed minority adoptions and current practices by adoption agencies in five large cities. Barriers identified by adoptive parents were poor communication skills of the workers, including not keeping contact, withholding information, or not making the applicant feel comfortable. About 20% (n = 8) of the families reported that they had been made to feel uncomfortable due to their race. Additionally, respondents identified overworked staff and unavailability of healthy children in public agencies as barriers.

Festinger and Pratt (2003) examined the retention of callers to a New York adoption hotline for two months in 2000 and 2001, with a total of 146 callers interviewed for the study. Of the participants who did not attend an orientation course following the initial call, 11.5% of respondents reported agency unresponsiveness or insufficient information as the reasons for not attending. When asked about general barriers to adopting a child from foster care, the primary concerns identified were the children's problems (21%), length of the process (18%), and the role of birth families (15%).

Adoptive applicants in a study by Katz (2005) expressed frustration with the initial phone call to the agency–ranging from getting no answer, leaving unreturned messages, and bouncing from one worker to the next before finding the appropriate person. With regard to homestudies required by some agencies in order to adopt, participants felt as though their workers were not listening to what they were saying, as well as inattentive to their preferences.

Adoption Timeframes and Costs

While there is an abundance of anecdotal information regarding how much time an adoption may take, there is a dearth of empirical evidence in the scholarly literature. Indeed, there are data tracking how long it takes for children to become adopted; however, none on how long it takes families, from starting the homestudy to finalization, to adopt a child. The American World Adoption Association (2006) states than an international adoption can be completed in nine to seventeen months. According to one public agency (State of Florida Department of Children and Families, 2006), the time it can take for a family to adopt a child from the foster care system can vary greatly. The process to become an approved adoptive parent includes attending a preparation course of ten weeks, with additional time to obtain local, state and federal background checks, current physical exam, and completion of a homestudy. This initial requirement can usually be completed in eight months. However, the time taken to have a child placed in the home and the adoption finalized was unavailable.

Katz (2005) conducted the largest study of attrition among prospective adoptive parents of children in foster care. The study was comprised of four different data collection and analysis efforts. According to the survey, financial reasons have made potential adoptive parents less likely to complete an adoption with the aforementioned agencies.

According to the National Adoption Information Clearinghouse (2006), the total cost of adopting varies greatly, depending on the agency/source selected, ranging from $0-$40,000. Foster care adoptions range from $0-$2,500; licensed private agency adoptions range from $5,000 to $40,000 + ; and inter-country adoptions ranging from $7000 to $30,000, depending on the country the child is adopted from. Adoptive parents can also encounter additional fees for travel, passport fees, visa processing fees, translation fees, or escorting fees if the parents do not travel but instead hire an individual to do so. Although somewhat dated, Berry, Barth, and Needell (1996) found that the mean cost of adoption for participants (n = 1008) in their study totaled $3751. Independent adoptions (n = 517) had the highest cost of $5766, private adoptions (n = 103) came in second with a cost of $5218, and lastly public agency adoptions (n = 388) averaged a cost of $645.1

Satisfaction with the Adoption Experience

Ninety percent (n = 35) of the minority families reported that they were very satisfied or satisfied with their last agency (Rodriguez & Meyer, 1990). Satisfaction with the agency selected for the 27 families who had completed an adoption was based on the ability to adopt the child they desired. Adoptive and waiting families also reported satisfaction due to a warm reception at intake and orientation, the presence of adoptive parents on staff, and the fact that it did not take many years to adopt (Rodriguez & Meyer, 1990). Forty one percent (n = 16) of the minority families had approached two or more agencies before selecting one (Rodriguez & Meyer, 1990). Experiences with private agencies were often negative. Nearly one-fifth of the families considered giving up on either the agency or adoption overall due to the high levels of dissatisfaction (Rodriguez & Meyer, 1990).

Berry, Barth and Needell (1996) surveyed adoptive parents who had filed for adoption in California between 1988 and 1989. Questionnaires were used to ascertain the overall preparation, support, and satisfaction of adoptive families in both agency and independent adoptions. Regardless of the differences in agency type, the vast majority of adoptive parents would recommend their adoption agency.

In the study by Katz (2005), participants tended to view the process favorably, with 99% agreeing or strongly agreeing on the training sessions provided by adoption agencies as being helpful with the preparation to adopt. Nine out of ten participants also stated that they would recommend the agency with which they worked to friends or relatives interested in adoption. However, approximately one in four participants did not feel as though the adoption worker provided an accurate estimate of the length of time it may take to have a child placed with them (25%) or advocated for them or encouraged them (23%). Furthermore, more than a third of the participants (35%) disagreed that the agency was actively trying to place a child with them.

The three areas outlined above (sources of consultation/information and possible bias, adoption timeframes and costs, and satisfaction with the adoption experience) illustrate the challenges often encountered on the road to becoming an adoptive parent. This study seeks to examine how these domains within the adoption process are similar or different across adoption type (international, private/domestic, and public child welfare) for the lesbian applicants in this sample. Factors will include the agencies consulted, costs of adoption, overall time for the adoption process, and perceived barriers encountered; and how the method of adoption (i.e., international, child welfare or private domestic) chosen by the respondents impact these outcomes.

METHODOLOGY

This study utilized a cross-sectional survey design. The survey was administered to gay and lesbian individuals and couples throughout the United States although, for this paper, only persons self-identifying as a lesbian will be included. The cross-sectional nature of the design does not allow for comparisons over time, but does allow the study to present a multi-dimensional perspective on these families' demographics, who they consulted with during the adoption process, how long it took to adopt their child, what costs were incurred, and, finally, their satisfaction with the overall adoption process. As noted above, each of these will be further examined across adoption types to help illustrate which avenues of adoption, for this sample, were most supportive.

Sample

To recruit participants, this study advertised through a variety of media in order to maximize the participation of individuals across the country. Newspaper ads were placed in several metropolitan gay and lesbian weekly newspapers, adoption magazines, gay parenting magazines, as well as a designated website. Additionally, flyers were distributed to both gay and lesbian and adoption organizations, and through a gay and lesbian adoptive parent listserv. The sample is non-random and therefore cannot be generalized to the larger gay and lesbian adoptive parent population, but rather the findings provide information only on the sample. A non-random sample was used because of the difficulty with gaining access to this population.

Data Collection Process

As was mentioned previously, the study recruited participants through a number of different media in order to reach the largest possible number of individuals and couples who had adopted a child. A 1-800 number and email address were created in order to provide participants with ways in which to contact the research staff. Once contact was initiated by the participants through either email or the phone, one of the researchers would contact the parent and would describe the purpose of the study, the procedures, and if they wanted to participate, the researcher obtained their address. A cover letter, consent form, and survey were sent to all participants who were interested in participating in the survey. Parents were encouraged to contact the researchers if they had any questions about the survey or the procedures. Two hundred and eighty-one surveys were sent to potential respondents. One hundred and eighty-three surveys were returned for an overall response rate of 65.1% which, according to Dillman (1978), constitutes a good response rate. Of these respondents, 96 self-identified as lesbian and are included in the analyses below.

Data Preparation

Following inspection of data for errors in entry and initial frequency distributions, missing values were replaced using the expectation-maximization method of imputation (Hill, 1997). This technique was selected for its capacity to employ a broad range of variables (rather than, for instance, sample means for a single variable) in the replacement of missing values. Given the sensitive nature of the topic, the occurrence of missing data was not unexpected. To determine if a variable could be kept and missing values imputed, the missing values had to be missing completely at random (MCAR). This condition is satisfied when a non-significant p-value is obtained using Little's chi-square test. If this assumption is met, "[both] complete cases . . . [and] EM . . . methods give consistent and unbiased estimates of correlations and covariances (Hill, 1997, p. 42). As such, for this sample, the Little's MCAR test obtained resulted in a Chi-Square = 5472.610 (df = 6454; p < 1.00) that indicates that the data are indeed MCAR (i.e., no identifiable pattern exists in the missing data). Lastly, because data are treated as continuous by the imputation program, the missing value estimations may fall outside of the given data range for variables using a Likert-type scale. In instances where this occurred, the value was transformed to represent the outer-most high/low value within the scale range.

Measures

The survey was a total of 28 pages (approximately 950 questions) that assessed a variety of domains. The domains included information on the demographics of the parent(s), child(ren), adopted child of focus (i.e., the oldest adopted child in the home), and the family, gay and lesbian community involvement, "out" status, adoption process and experiences, the adoption timeline, adoption costs and subsidy, the adopted child of focus' pre- and post-adoptive experiences, overall adoption experience, satisfaction with services, family dynamics, social support, parent and adopted child of focus relationship, the adopted child of focus' birth family, and several psychometric assessment instruments. While all of these areas were included in the survey, only those focusing on the adoption process will be presented in this paper.

Included in the larger survey were eight questions asking parents about their level of satisfaction with the adoption social worker's[2] services provided when adopting the index child. This satisfaction scale has been used with other adoptive samples and exhibited acceptable reliability and validity (Nalavany, 2006). The mean score of these items will be used in the analyses rather than using a single item as an indicator, as a composite score shares more of its variance with the purported concept and is more statistically reliable than a single item indicator (Little, Cunningham, Shahar, & Wildaman, 2002). Reliability and validity analyses were undertaken to identify any potential weak items that may obscure the scale's potential usefulness. Utilizing a confirmatory factor analysis, all items were shown to load equal to or greater than .60, and in the desired direction. The satisfaction scores for social work support at adoption were in the 'somewhat satisfied' range of satisfaction (M = 3.91; SD = .95) and had an excellent alpha of .91. Potentially weak items were assessed based on the estimated "alpha if deleted" values using SPSS software. Based on this assessment, no weak items were found. Therefore, no modifications were made to this measure.

FINDINGS

Adoptive Parent Demographics

The data in Table 1 provide basic information on the 96 lesbian adoptive parents who completed the survey. As noted in the table, almost 93% of respondents were partnered. As such, while some families were able to adopt jointly, due to the laws in most states most of the partnered respondents were not able to adopt as a couple. Nevertheless, it is recognized that these families function as such, and most indicated this status on the survey when asked about their relationship with the child. Most, if not already related to the child via birth, checked the 'would be if I could be' adoptive parent. As such, the oldest parent was asked to complete Parent #1 information, and the younger one was asked to complete Parent #2 information. This recognized that even though only one may be legally recognized as the adoptive parent, both parents were of value and interest to the study.

TABLE 1. Adoptive Parent Characteristics

Question	Distribution	
	Parent #1	Parent #2
Age	45.53 (6.42)	41.12 (7.44)
Race/Ethnicity		
Caucasian	93.8	87.6
Hispanic	3.1	5.6
African American	2.1	1.1
Other	1.0	5.6
Education		
High School/GED	3.1	--
Some college or AA Degree	13.5	19.1
Bachelors degree	28.1	30.3
Masters degree	39.6	34.8
Doctoral degree	15.6	15.7
Employment		
Stay-At-Home Parent	12.5	21.3
Employed	87.5	78.7
Religion		
Christian	27.1	24.7
Unitarian	15.6	18.0
Jewish	10.4	6.7
Non-specific/spiritual	18.8	31.5
Other	28.1	19.1
Partnered (Yes)	92.7	
Number of Years Partnered	10.76 (6.39)	
Total Household Income	$95,028 ($55,476)	
Type of Community where individual/couple reside		
Large urban	37.5	
Small urban	17.7	
Suburban	31.3	
Rural	13.5	
Child Adopted		
Private-International	33.3	
Public-Child Welfare	27.1	
Private-Domestic	39.6	

NOTE: Mean (SD); All other numbers=Valid Percent

The parents' ages ranged from 29 years old to 64 years old, with the mean age of Parent #1 being 45.53 years old (sd = 6.42 years) and the average age of Parent #2 being 41.12 years old (sd = 7.44 years). The ethnicity of the sample was predominately Caucasian (93.8% Parent #1; 87.6% Parent #2). Overall, the sample was highly educated with over 80% of the sample having at least a Bachelor's degree. Likewise, the vast majority of the parents were employed full time. The religious background of the parents was fairly diverse, with over one-fourth of Parent #1 indicating that she was Christian. A similar finding was present for Parent #2, with almost 24% indicating that she was Christian. As mentioned previously, slightly over 92% of the sample were partnered and had been for an average of almost 11 years, ranging from 1 to 30 years. The total household annual income ranged from $20,000 to $400,000 with an average yearly income of $95,028 with a standard deviation of $55,476. Lastly, participants were asked to identify the type of community in which they resided; over one-third (37.5%) indicated that they resided in a large urban area, whereas 17.7% indicated that they lived in a small urban area. Slightly less than one-third (31.3%) indicated living in a suburban area, and only 13.5% indicated that they lived in a rural area.

The breakdown of the sources from which their children were adopted was almost evenly divided across international (33.3%), child welfare (39.6%) and private domestic adoptions (27.1%). Using Chi-Square and ANOVAs where appropriate, demographic data were examined across these three groups to determine if any significant differences exist. Due to the lack of empirical literature regarding such adoptive families, no specific a priori hypotheses were made regarding variable associations across adoption type. Results indicated that no significant differences across adoption types were observed for this sample's demographic responses. As such, it appears that all three groups of lesbian adoptive parents within this sample are, at least on the variables collected, demographically similar.

Sources of Consultation/Information and Possible Bias

The next section, as shown in Table 2, identifies the sources the prospective adoptive parents in this sample approached when contemplating adoption. Numerous sources were explored to see if they had been approached, and, if so, how helpful they were in supporting the adoption. To test if any significant differences exist across adoption types for the lesbian adoptive parents in this sample, ANOVAs were used as appropriate. Again, due to the lack of empirical evidence on this sample, no a priori hypotheses were made regarding which sources of information were used most often, or were most helpful, by adoption type.

For the full sample, adoption agencies were contacted for information when considering adoption the vast majority of the time (85.4%). When contacted, they appeared to be helpful/very helpful over 75% of the time. This source appeared to be equally helpful across adoption types, with no significant differences noted. Attorneys were contacted, on average, slightly less than half of the time when gathering information; however, lesbian parents adopting privately from domestic sources did so significantly more often (76% of the time) than the other two groups ($F = 3.052, p < .001$).[3] Nevertheless, when contacting an at-

TABLE 2. Sources of Consultation/Information and Possible Bias

Question	Yes		Helpful?			
		NVH	NH	M	H	VH
Did you consult an:						
Adoption agency?	85.4	6.1	8.5	9.8	31.7	43.9
Attorney?	44.8	11.6	14.0	9.3	39.5	25.6
Social worker?	56.3	13.0	9.3	16.7	29.8	31.5
Family?	66.7	6.3	14.1	40.6	20.3	18.8
Friends?	85.4	3.3	10.9	27.2	30.4	28.3
On-line sources?	61.5	5.8	14.5	17.4	33.3	29.0
Adoption books?	77.1	1.4	14.9	35.1	29.7	18.9
Non-LGBT adoptive parents?	50.0	2.1	6.3	14.6	47.9	29.2
LGBT adoptive parents?	66.7	1.6	7.8	15.6	35.9	39.1
Do you believe that you experienced bias or discrimination from:						
Attorney?	4.2					
Judge?	13.5					
Social worker?	5.2					
Adoption agency staff?	10.4					
Other agency professionals?	25.0					
Birth family?	6.3					

NOTE: All numbers=Valid Percent; NVH=Not Very Helpful; NH=Not Helpful; M=Mixed; H=Helpful; VH=Very Helpful

torney, most respondents felt that it was helpful/very helpful (65.1%). The last formal information source, social workers, showed no significant differences across adoption types for either contact or helpfulness. Slightly over half of the sample approached them, and, of those, approximately 60% found the information obtained helpful/very helpful.

Family was consulted about the adoption two-thirds of the time; however, they were not found to be very helpful. In fact, less than half (39.1%) of all lesbian adoptive parents reported their families as helpful/very helpful. Slightly more (40.6%) found this source somewhat mixed in its level of helpfulness. Friends, on the other hand, were consulted 85.4% of the time. When approached, the level of helpfulness varied significantly across adoption types. Persons adopting from a private domestic source found friends significantly more helpful ($\alpha = 4.14$, sd = .96) than did persons adopting from the child welfare system ($\alpha = 3.19$, sd = 1.02); although neither group was significantly different from the international adoption cohort ($\alpha = 3.60$, sd = 1.13) ($F = 6.490$, $p < .002$).

The lesbian adoptive parents in this sample searched for and consulted with online sources 61.5% of the time; with most (62.3%) finding the information helpful/very helpful. Adoption books were consulted slightly more than three-fourths of the time (77.1%); however, less than half of the respondents (48.6%) found the information obtained therein as either helpful or very helpful. In fact, the most frequently cited response was mixed (35.1%). No significant differences were found across adoption types for either online sources or adoption texts.

Lastly, respondents were asked about their interactions with other adoptive parents during their adoption process. Only half of the respondents consulted with non-LGBT adoptive parents. However, of those that did, they found this to be the most helpful source of information—with 77.1% finding non-LGBT adoptive parents helpful or very helpful. This level of helpfulness spanned all adoption types, with no significant differences noted. Other LGBT adoptive parents were also consulted by 66.7% of the lesbian respondents. This, too, was also found to be helpful/very helpful (75.0%); although public child welfare adopters found this to be significantly less helpful than their counterparts.

Some level of bias or discrimination was reported from all sources; although all were relatively low (only other agency professionals reached as high as 25%). Birth families were experienced as a source of bias or discrimination significantly more for lesbians adopting from the child welfare system (15% of the time vs. 5% for private domestic and none for international sources) ($F = 3.044, p < .05$).

Adoption Timeframes and Costs

Table 3 identifies the average length of time families spent within each phase of the adoption process, as well as the costs associated with various aspects of adopting a child. ANOVAs were utilized to examine the length of time taken within each step across adoption types. As discussed previously, there were no a priori assumptions made regarding differences across types. Similar calculations were conducted for the cost data collected.

The average time taken from thinking about the adoption to finalization was approximately 3 years, with no significant differences found across adoption types. However, within the overall adoption process there were three steps in which one group outpaced another: finishing the course to homestudy approval; child presented to placement; and placement to finalization. Those parents adopting from a private domestic source took significantly longer ($M = .38$ years, sd = .36 years) from course completion to homestudy approval than did persons adopting from the child welfare system ($M = .19$ years, sd = .19 years) although neither group was significantly different from the international adoption cohort ($M = .26$ years, sd = .28 years) ($F = 3.418, p < .037$). Con-

TABLE 3. Adoption Timeframes and Costs

Question	Distribution
Timing of Adoption Process Steps (in years)	
Average time from thinking to starting course	1.29 (1.75)
Average time from starting to finishing course	.23 (.30)
Average time from finishing course to homestudy approval	.29 (.30)
Average time from homestudy approval to child presented	.40 (.42)
Average time from child presented to placed	.16 (.24)
Average time from child placed to adoption finalized	.74 (.89)
Average total time	3.12 (2.14)
How satisfied were you with the accuracy of the timeline given for your adoption?	
Very dissatisfied	8.3
Somewhat dissatisfied	6.3
Mixed	26.0
Somewhat satisfied	28.1
Very satisfied	31.3
Cost of Adoption (in dollars)	
Travel	$1,355 ($1,950)
Lawyer	$1,967 ($3,309)
Homestudy	$990 ($1,220)
Medical-Birth Mother	$537 ($1,922)
Medical-Child	$795 ($4,409)
Other	$8,151 ($37,416)
Average total cost	$13,797 ($42,555)
How satisfied were you with the accuracy, explanation and breakdown of the expenses of your adoption?	
Very dissatisfied	3.1
Somewhat dissatisfied	7.3
Mixed	14.6
Somewhat satisfied	30.2
Very satisfied	44.8

NOTE: Mean (SD); All other numbers=Valid Percent

versely, those parents adopting from a private domestic source took significantly less time ($M = .08$ years, sd = .14 years) from having the child presented for consideration to when the child was placed with the family than did persons adopting internationally ($M = .26$ years, sd = .25 years) although neither group was significantly different from the child welfare cohort ($M = .18$ years, sd = .31 years) ($F = 5.074$, $p < .008$). Lastly, international adoptions took significantly less time from placement to finalization ($M = .28$ years, sd = .51 years) than did persons adopting from either private domestic sources or the child welfare system ($M = .84$, sd = .95 years and $M = 1.18$ years, sd = .95 years, respectively) ($F = 8.808$, $p < .001$).

Overall, the majority of respondents (59.4%) were generally satisfied with the accuracy of the timeline provided. However, significant differences were noted across cohorts ($F = 4.443$, $p < .014$). Lesbian parents adopting from the child welfare system were significantly less satisfied with the projected versus actual time frames (only 42.3% responded as either somewhat or very satisfied) than were persons adopting from private domestic sources (73.6% were somewhat or very satisfied). There was no significant difference between either and international adoptions (56.3% were somewhat or very satisfied).

There were no significant cost differences within three specific categories: birth mother's medical expenses, adopted child's medical expenses, or other expenses. However, there were significant differences noted for each of the other categories, including the overall total cost. Lesbian parents adopting internationally bore a significantly higher amount of travel costs ($M = \$2,948$, sd = \$2,456$) than did either persons adopting from the child welfare system or from private domestic sources ($M = \$304$, sd = \$712$ and $M = \$733$, sd = \$1,000$, respectively) ($F = 24.477$, $p < .001$). The cost of hiring an attorney was most expensive for parents adopting internationally ($M = \$3,599$, sd = \$4,693$), with parents adopting privately from domestic agencies at about half as much ($M = \$1,767$, sd = \$2,225$); although there was no significant difference between the two. A significant difference was found between persons adopting internationally and via the child welfare system ($M = \$250$, sd = \$660$) ($F = 8.667$, $p < .001$).

Homestudy costs varied widely by adoption type, with each adoption venue being significantly different from the other ($F = 16.150$, $p < .001$). Homestudy costs associated with adopting a child from the child welfare system averaged \$124 (sd = \$317). Private domestic adoptions was significantly higher ($M = \$971$, sd = \$1,052$), with homestudies completed for applicants adopting internationally significantly higher still ($M = \$1,718$, sd = \$1,409$). Lastly, the total cost of the adoption was, on average, \$13,797. Significant cost differences were found, with international adoptions costing significantly more ($M = \$30,412$, sd = \$70,685$) than did those from the child welfare system ($M = \$1,340$, sd = \$2,611$) although neither group was significantly different from private domestic adoptions ($M = \$8,330$, sd = \$8,967$) ($F = 4.121$, $p < .008$).

Satisfaction with the Adoption Experience

As noted previously, eight questions regarding the adoptive parent's level of satisfaction on various criteria were gathered. As illustrated in Table 4, adoptive parents clearly indicated that they were somewhat/very satisfied (73.0%) with the social worker's inclusion of the parents in setting goals. The majority of adoptive parents were also somewhat/very satisfied with the social worker's responsiveness

TABLE 4. Satisfaction with the Adoption Experience

Question	Distribution				
	VD	SD	M	SS	VS
How satisfied were you with your adoption social worker's level of involving you (and your partner, if applicable) in setting goals?	6.3	8.3	12.5	29.2	43.8
How satisfied were you with your adoption social worker's responsiveness to your questions and concerns?	5.2	4.2	11.5	24.0	55.2
How satisfied were you with your adoption social worker's knowledge of clinical adoption-related issues?	3.1	6.3	24.0	24.0	42.7
How satisfied were you with your adoption social worker's handling of any problems experienced?	9.4	9.4	13.5	28.1	39.6
How satisfied were you with your adoption social worker's level of concern for the ADOPTED CHILD OF FOCUS?	7.3	4.2	7.3	21.9	59.4
How satisfied were you with your adoption social worker's level of concern for your individual family?	7.3	3.1	15.6	24.0	50.0
How satisfied were you with the accuracy of the timeline given for your adoption?	8.3	6.3	26.0	28.1	31.3
How satisfied were you with the quality and quantity of the medical information you received on the ADOPTED CHILD OF FOCUS?	13.5	7.3	27.1	26.0	26.0
Satisfaction with Adoption Process			3.91 (.95)		

NOTE: Mean (SD); All other numbers=Valid Percent; VD=Very Dissatisfied; SD=Somewhat Dissatisfied; M=Mixed; SS=Somewhat Satisfied; VS=Very Satisfied

(79.2%), knowledge of adoption issues (66.7%), handling of any problems (67.7%), level of concern for the child (81.3%), and adoptive family (74.0%).

Two items were found to have significant differences across adoption cohorts–the accuracy of the timeline given (which was discussed above), and the quality and quantity of medical information received. While slightly more than half (52.0%) of the adoptive parents were somewhat/very satisfied with the quantity and quality of the medical information received on their adopted child, significant differences were found between international and private domestic adoptions; with international adoptions the least satisfied (31.3% were somewhat/very satisfied). Those from private domestic sources were the most satisfied (68.4% were somewhat/very satisfied). Neither group was significantly different from child welfare adoptions (53.9% were somewhat/very satisfied) ($F = 4.464$, $p < .014$).

DISCUSSION

The lesbian respondents in this sample had all successfully adopted a child from any one of three avenues, and were closely split in the frequency of matches via international, private domestic, or public child welfare sources. As they traveled this road to become adoptive parents, various sources of information were consulted, with varying levels of helpfulness and bias, sometimes experienced differentially across adoption types. Similar to the findings of Brodzinsky, Patterson and Vaziri (2002) where agencies were found to be generally open to working with lesbian (or gay) prospective adoptive parents, the lesbian respondents in this sample felt that the agencies they contacted were overwhelmingly helpful. Although there was some variation across adoption types, other formal sources of information were also found to be helpful. Given the heterosexist opinions held by some child welfare workers (Ryan, 2000; Taylor, 1998), it is encouraging to see that the experiences of this sample of lesbian adoptive parents was generally positive.

These findings help to illustrate to other lesbians wishing to adopt where some potentially helpful sources of information exist, as well as some possible sources of bias or discrimination. This information may also help adoption professionals working with such clients to support them as they, for example, discuss the possible adoption with family members who, as experienced by several respondents in this sample, may not be very helpful in the adoption process. In addition, irrespective of the venue through which they adopted (international, private/domestic, or public child welfare), all women reported some level of perceived bias (with 10% or more women reporting bias in three of the categories listed in Table 2). As such, it is imperative that professional and agency policies be created and enforced to foster an atmosphere of openness–with educational and other opportunities made available to teach adoption professionals about this population.

As noted above, there is much known about how long it takes children to go through the process of adoption–from removal from the birth family to finalization with the adoptive family, especially for children adopted from the foster care system. However, there is virtually no empirical evidence on the adoptive parents' path through this process. Overall, the steps in the adoption process are very similar across adoption types, with some steps being significantly shorter or longer for some groups. Nevertheless, from the point of considering adoption to finalization, the overall timeline was not significantly different for the parents in this sample. This is an important consideration for many prospective adoptive parents, and, if time is equivalent across groups, as it was for this sample, this information may help them make the most appropriate choice for their individual circumstance. Conversely, the costs associated with adopting their child varied significantly and may prove to be a more relevant consideration (among many other important factors). In general, the findings reported for the lesbian adoptive parents in this sample are consistent with the limited data reported in the literature (NAIC, 2006; Berry, Barth & Needell, 1996).

The lesbian adoptive parents in this sample were, on average, somewhat satisfied with their overall adoption experience, with each satisfaction scale item having the majority of the full sample rating it as being somewhat/very satisfied. These findings are consistent with the limited literature available, although some points may need continued attention. These include the accuracy of the timelines provided, as well as the quality and quantity of medical information received, especially from persons adopting internationally. Adoption practitioners should make every effort to convey timely and accurate information to aid lesbian adoptive parents (indeed, all adoptive parents) through this often challenging life transition. A satisfactory relationship is not only important in facilitating the adoption, but in ensuring its continued success–as families having a strained relationship with adoption professionals may not feel comfortable asking for help and may feel like failures; thus increasing the risk of an adoption disruption, displacement or dissolutionment (Ryan, Glover & Cash, 2006).

As with all studies, this one contained some limitations. Of primary concern is that the convenience sample may introduce selection bias. It is possible that participants were only those families who believed that they had positive encounters and had strengths to discuss, thus leaving out families who may have had negative pre-adoption experiences. In addition, all of the results are based on self-report and these parents may have wanted to portray their experience in the most positive light. There was no control or comparison group. Thus, we can talk about the experiences of these lesbian adoptive parents' transition to adoptive parenthood, but we cannot compare these findings to non-lesbian adoptive parents or, indeed, to any group beyond this sample. Lastly, these data were collected cross-sectionally and they do not permit us to understand the dynamics of life in these and other adoptive families. One would have to recruit families as they begin the adoption process and follow them throughout to gain a complete understanding of how these factors interplay as they become adoptive parents. However, it should be noted that the limitations above are not unique to research on lesbian-(or gay) headed adoptive families, and similar longitudinal/developmental research is needed on all adoptive family forms.

Nevertheless, despite these limitations, the study, utilizing the largest sample of lesbian adoptive parents to date, was able to illustrate part of the process that lesbians travel on the road to becoming adoptive parents. In fact, three roads could be traveled–and these were compared and contrasted to further demonstrate this experience in the hopes of informing other lesbians wishing to adopt, as well as adoption professionals, of areas that may need improvement as adoptive family forms continue to become more diverse. While there is a growing body of literature describing gay and lesbian adoptive experiences, it is also clear that much more empirical work is needed to gain a complete understanding of adoptions in general, as well as adoptive gay and lesbian parents and their children in particular. Future research should address some of the current gaps by obtaining a large representative sample, incorporating a comparison group of non-gay/lesbian adoptive parents, and, independent of parental reporting, collecting data from adoptive children on how they grow and develop within such families. While there is no evidence that such adoptions are harmful in any way, and growing evidence that such placements are as loving and supportive as adoptive families in general, more rigorous research will enable adoption practitioners and policy-makers to be more responsive and supportive to the needs of this all too often hidden adoptive family form.

NOTES

1. These cost data are taken directly from the article and have not been adjusted for inflation.

2. The survey question asked about the satisfaction with the *adoption social worker's* services; however, it is recognized that professionally trained social workers only make up a portion of persons providing social work-type adoption services.

3. Tukey, Scheffe and Bonferroni post hoc tests were utilized, where, to be conservative, a minimum of two out of three must confirm the significant difference. This standard is used throughout the paper.

REFERENCES

American Academy of Child and Adolescent Psychiatry. (1999). Policy statement: Gay, lesbian and bisexual parents. Retrieved February 25, 2006 from http://www.aacap.org/publications/policy/ps46.htm.

American Academy of Pediatrics. (2002). *Coparent or second-parent adoption by same-sex parents.* Retrieved February 25, 2006 from http://www.aap.org/policy/020008.html.

American Psychiatric Association. (1986). Position statement on discrimination in selection of foster parents. *American Journal of Psychiatry, 143,* 1506.

American Psychoanalytic Association. (2002). *Position statement on gay and lesbian parenting.* Retrieved February 25, 2006 from http://apsa-co.org/ctf/cgli/parenting.htm

American Psychological Association. (1975). *Policy statements on lesbian, gay, and bisexual concerns: Discrimination against homosexuals.* Retrieved February 25, 2006 from http://www.apa.org/pi/lgbpolicy/child.html.

American Psychological Association. (1976). *Policy statements on lesbian, gay, and bisexual concerns: Child custody or placement.* Retrieved February 25, 2006 from http://www.apa.org/pi/lgbpolicy/against.html.

American World Adoption Association. (2006). *Frequently asked questions.* Retrieved February 25, 2006 from http://www.awaa.org/faq/#anchor9.

Appell, A. (2003). Recent developments in lesbian and gay adoption law. *Adoption Quarterly, 7*(1), 73-84.

Bausch, R., & Serpe, R. (1999). Recruiting Mexican American parents. *Child Welfare, 78,* 693-716.

Berry, M., Barth, R., & Needell, B. (1996). Preparation, support, and satisfaction of adoptive families in agency and independent adoptions. *Child & Adolescent Social Work Journal, 13*(2), 157-183.

Black, D., Gates, G., Sanders, S., & Taylor, L. (2000). Demographics of the gay and lesbian population in the U.S.: Evidence from available systematic data sources. *Demography, 37,* 139-154.

Brodzinsky, D., Patterson, C., & Vaziri, M. (2002). Adoption agency perspectives on lesbian and gay prospective parents: A national study. *Adoption Quarterly, 5*(3), 5-23.

Child Welfare League of America. (2006). *National Data Analysis System.* Retrieved January 11, 2006 from http://ndas.cwla.org.

Dillman, D. A. (2000). *Mail and internet surveys: The tailored design method* (2nd ed.). Toronto: John Wiley & Sons.

Festinger, T., & Pratt, R. (2003). Retaining interest: A look at New York City's recruitment of adoptive parents for waiting children.

Hill, M. (1997). *SPSS missing values analysis 7.5.* Chicago, IL., SPSS Inc.

Katz, J. (2005). *Listening to parents: Overcoming barriers to the adoption of children from foster care.* New York: Evan B. Donaldson Adoption Institute.

Kreider, R. (2003) Adopted children and stepchildren. Census 2000 Special Reports. U.S. Census Bureau.

Little, T. D., Cunningham, W. A., Shahar, G., & Wildaman, K. F. (2002). To parcel or not to parcel: Exploring the question, weighing the merits. *Structural Equation Modeling, 9,* 151-173.

Nalavany, B. (2006). *The impact of preadoptive childhood sexual abuse on adopted boys.* Unpublished manuscript: Tallahassee, FL.

National Association of Social Workers. (2000). *Code of ethics of the National Association of Social Workers* (Section 4.02). Retrieved February 25, 2006 from http://www.naswdc.org/pubs/code/default.htm.

North American Council on Adoptable Children. (2002). *Gay and lesbian adoptions and foster care.* Retrieved February 25, 2006 from http://www.nacac.org/pub_statements.html#gay.

Rodriguez, P. & Meyer, A. (1990). Minority adoptions and agency practices. *Social Work, 35,* 528-531.

Rothman, J., Damron-Rodriquez, J., & Shenassa, E. (1994). Systematic research synthesis: Conceptual integration methods of meta-analysis. In J. Rothman & E. J. Thomas (Eds.), *Intervention research: Design and development for human service* (pp. 133-160). New York: Haworth.

Ryan, S. (In Press). Adoptive Families Headed by Gay Men and Lesbians. In V. Bullough and K. Stolley (Eds.), *A Historical and Cross-Cultural Encyclopedia of Adoption.* Westport, CT: Greenwood Press.

Ryan, S. (2000). Examining social workers' placement recommendations of children with gay and lesbian adoptive parents. *Families in Society,* 81, 517-528.

Ryan, S., Bedard, L., & Gertz, M. (2004). Florida's gay adoption ban: What do Floridians think? *Journal of Law and Public Policy,* 15, 261-284.

Ryan, S., Glover, A., & Cash, S. (2006). Conceptual mapping the challenges faced by adoptive parents in utilizing post-placement services. In M. Dore (Ed.), *The Post-Adoption Experience: Adoptive Families' Service Needs and Service Outcomes (pp. 251-282).* Washington, DC: Child Welfare League of America.

Ryan, S., Pearlmutter, S., & Groza, V. (2004). Coming out of the closet: Opening agencies to gay and lesbian adoptive parents. *Social work, 49*(1), 85-95.

Shelley-Sireci, L., Ciano-Boyce, C. (2002). Becoming lesbian adoptive parents: An exploratory study of lesbian adoptive, lesbian birth, and heterosexual adoptive parents. *Adoption Quarterly, 6*(1), 33-43.

State of Florida Department of Children and Families. (2006). *Frequently asked questions about the adoption program.* Retrieved March 11, 2006, from http://www.dcf.state.fl.us/adoption/faq.shtml.

Taylor, M. (1998). Attitudes of social workers toward gay and lesbian adoption. Unpublished master's thesis, California State University, Long Beach. (UMI No. 1390139, MAI 36/05, p. 1276).

Time. (2006, March 20). Notebook. *Author, 167*(12), p. 30

Lesbian Parents and Work: Stressors and Supports for the Work-Family Interface

Lucy R. Mercier

In American society, work has value beyond providing subsistence for one's family. For many people, work is intrinsically linked to identity. Choosing an occupation, working toward a career goal, and surviving transitions in the workplace involve changes in self-presentation, social status, and relationship patterns. Mothers who leave paid employment to stay home with children report that they leave behind important sources of social support and have less-robust self-definition (Mercier & Harold, 2001).

In addition, gender remains a fundamental element in structuring perceptions of both work and family. The past half-century has seen huge changes in work and family lives, but many contemporary family researchers report that their respondents still organize their perceptions of family life around traditional ideas of sex and gender (Smith & Beaujot, 1999). That is, many people continue to assume, as part of the normal social order, that families should include men who work to support themselves and their families, while women's first responsibilities lie with their families, especially their children.

Similarly, much of existing family theory assumes that families are anchored by heterosexual couples, whose production of offspring starts the cycle of normal family development (e.g. Parsons & Bales, 1955). When it comes to working outside the home for financial support, this normative model of family development relies heavily on the maintenance of traditional gender roles and gendered expressions of work (male provider / female homemaker), and any variance from the prescribed arrangement of the family-career relationship is thought to result in work-family role overloads (Voydanoff,1987).

For most American women, being partnered does not seem to be correlated with long-term absence from the workplace. Studies of heterosexual-parent families show that the majority include two workers. As many as 80% of women who were employed before childbirth return to work within 12 months of their babies' births (Gornick & Meyers, 2001), and 3/4 of preschoolers have mothers who work outside the home (Klerman & Leibowitz, 1990).

In response to the changing patterns of work-family interactions, workplace programs such as support for dependent care, flexible work schedules, paid family leave, short-term counseling, and employee wellness education programs are on the rise (Singleton, 2000). But employees' use of these programs depends on the workplace milieu as well as the types of family needs being experienced (Fredriksen-Goldsen & Scharlach, 2001). The research described in this paper attempted to explore and describe the work-family situations of lesbian parents by addressing the following questions: How is the work-family intersection experienced in lesbian parent families? What are the most important issues for lesbian parents who work outside the home? What are the major sources of stress and support in the workplace for lesbian-headed households?

This paper reports on these data related to the work-family issues experienced by lesbian parents. The data were gathered in a qualitative study of lesbian parent families in one Midwestern state. The research project from which these data were taken was a larger, in-depth exploration of lesbian parents' relationships within their households, and between their households and the organizations and institutions around them. To provide background, an overview of the larger study's methodology and sampling is presented, but the focus of this paper is on the themes and issues identified by the study respondents as important to them in their work lives. Giving attention to the families' strategies for managing the work-family relationship should provide important information for social service providers who work with these families.

Descriptive research on the statistical relevance of sexual orientation in terms of oppression is difficult to accomplish because of the reluctance of research subjects to identify themselves. However, gay men and lesbians experience rejection by families of origin and important sources of interpersonal support, employment discrimination, denial of certain employment-related benefits (e.g. domestic partner programs and family leave), barriers to legally-recognized marriage (and thus all the federal and state benefits that marriage confers), threats to child custody, and increased risk of anti-gay violence (Cahill, Ellen & Tobias, 2003; Harvard Law Review, 1990). In addition to these rather concrete issues, lesbians and gay men have long reported that social stigmatization and the fear of subtler forms of discrimination or rejection negatively impact the quality of their lives (McDonald & Steinhorn, 1993). This study rested on the assumption that lesbians are challenged by social, economic, and interpersonal factors and that these conditions influence their experiences as members of families. Rather than focusing on problems, however, I hoped that the nature of the research design would yield data that reflects both obstacles and opportunities in the respondents' families and social interactions.

Since the 1970's, research has emphasized the strengths of lesbian respondents by examining their social behavior, intimate relationships, political and occupational roles, sexual norms, and families of origin. In the last decades of the 20th century, studies that focused on adolescence, adulthood, midlife, and aging collected data on the spectrum of experiences and issues encountered by lesbians (Laird, 1994; Tully, 1995). In contrast to the early deficit-driven research on etiology and psychological functioning, these studies focused on the role of the helping professional in assisting lesbians to manage the unique stressors of living as an oppressed minority and paid particular attention to the unique structures and relationships formed in various lesbian parent families (Parks, 1998).

It is important to understand the experiences of lesbians in the social world; the world of work is an integral part of every parent's social world, including most lesbian parents. Only when understanding is achieved is it possible to move into planning for effective service and for social change. The principles and methods of feminist qualitative research, which guided this project, offer an opportunity to introduce the perspectives of lesbian parents themselves into the body of family research, even though sampling limitations make generalization of results impossible.

METHOD

Methods used in data collection and analysis for this study were informed by principles of feminist epistemology, including the idea that creating social change is an integral part of the research process (Fonow & Cook, 1991). Because a primary motivation of the research was to better understand the experiences of the respondents from their own perspectives, an interactive model of data analysis utilized both deductive and inductive approaches in order to produce highly-detailed descriptive data (Strauss & Corbin, 1990). The study was approved by the human subjects committee of a major research university.

This study used a non-representative sample of lesbian parents, who were recruited using a modified snowball sampling method. Clusters of potential participants were identified and contacted for the purpose of completing questionnaires that included demographic and background information on the participants and their families. From the 125 completed questionnaires, 102 women (81.6%) included contact information indicating willingness to participate in face-to-face interviews. From this pool, a sub-sample of 21 lesbian parents was selected. As with other studies of lesbian parents (see Demo & Allen, 1996), the larger sample was skewed toward upper-income, university-educated women, although other characteristics were represented as well. Therefore, the sub-sample was deliberately chosen to maximize diversity in terms of race, income, education, employment, age of parents and children, and methods of family formation.

The 21 women interviewed represented 15 families. All but one of the participants were partnered, with relationships ranging in length from a few months to nearly 20 years. Children in these families ranged in age from 6 months to 17 years old. While most of the women were white, 3 (14%) were African American. The children, as a group, were more racially diverse than their parents, with 50% being identified as children of color.

The face-to-face, semi-structured interviews took place in participants' homes or workplaces (n = 16), although some respondents (n = 5) were seen in the interviewers' office for reasons of confidentiality or convenience. Interviews lasted from one to two hours, on average. The interview protocol was adapted from a study of heterosexual-parent families (Harold, Mercier, & Colarossi, 1997), with new interview questions developed from the literature on lesbian parent families and from the questionnaire responses. Interviews focused on family relationships with the social environment, and included queries specifically about the relationships between members of the respondent's household and paid employment. Interviewees were asked to describe their feelings about work, describing sources of stress and support, and to discuss the strategies they used for managing their interactions with the world of work.

Researchers took extensive notes during the interview sessions. Interviewers' notes included content summaries, verbatim statements, notes on non-verbal communication, and key words or phrases used in each interview. Notes were discussed and checked with respondents throughout the interviews.

Analysis of the narrative data in this study used an interactive model, in which both deductive and inductive approaches were used to produce richly detailed, descriptive data. First, all interview data relating to the relationship between the respondents' families and work were identified and coded. From this larger class of data, categories were derived, based on the respondents' comments as well as themes suggested from the literature on work and family. Thus, respondents' ideas were privileged, in keeping with the study's commitment to feminist research methods. Results of the analysis are reported using pseudonyms and disguised personal descriptions in order to retain the unique character of the respondents, whenever possible without violating confidentiality.

RESULTS

Family employment arrangements ranged from a single woman with a part-time job to families with two full-time workers. Of the 15 households represented by interviewees, all contained at least one adult worker. Most (80%) of the families had two incomes, but only a third of the households had two full-time workers. The work lives of the participant families were complex. Twelve (57%) of the women interviewed worked full-time. Six others (29%) identified themselves as part-time workers. Three of the women interviewed (14%) were self-employed or entrepreneurs, and a total of seven families (47%) included adult students. Three respondents did not receive any wages because they were full-time care givers to their children. Household income level, of course, varied accordingly.

Each respondent was asked to characterize the type of relationship between her household and employment. Interviewees who lived in a household with two incomes were asked to provide data on their own work and on their partner's work. Respondents were shown a key with relationship types listed, from which they could select. The relationship types listed included: non-interactive (indicating no relationship between the workplace and the respondent's family members); strong/ positive; stressful / negative; tenuous / strained; and change in relationship (with a prompt for respondents to describe the change). Seventy percent (n = 14) of household-employment relationships were characterized as "strong / positive" for respondent's work. In addition, one respondent who identified the household-work relationship as a "change in relationship" added that the changes were very positive. Two women labeled their household-employment relationship as "stressful / negative." Two others said that the relationship was "tenuous / strained." Only one respondent indicated that her employment was "non-interactive" with her household. Respondents were also asked to rate their satisfaction with the household-respondent's work relationship on a 7-point scale, with higher values corresponding with greater levels of satisfaction. Results ranged from two to seven, and mean satisfaction was 5.67 (SD = 1.37).

Results for partner's work were remarkably similar. Sixty-five percent (n = 13) of partner's work relationships were labeled as "strong / positive." Again, a single respondent identified the household-work relationship as a "change in relationship" and indicated that work was "getting more positive." One woman labeled the household-partner's work relationship as "stressful / negative," and two said it was "tenuous

/ strained." Another three respondents said that their households were "non-interactive" with partners' work. Respondents' satisfaction with the relationship between their family and partners' work ranged from three to seven on the 7-point scale. The mean was 5.41 (SD = 1.58).

Overall, employed respondents held jobs that were above average in salary and prestige, which may account for some of their positive perceptions of the interactions between households and work. Interestingly, all household-work relationships identified as "stressful / negative" referred to respondents' or partners' jobs in the social service field. Household-work relationships characterized as "tenuous / strained" were accompanied by descriptions of jobs that interfered with workers' time and energy for the family. Non-interactive' relationships occurred only in blended families. That is, respondents only reported no relationship between their work and their family in cases where the respondents' current family consisted of children from a previous union with another male or female partner.

Analysis of the narrative data allowed a fuller picture of the respondents' relationships with work to emerge. The following sections provide details about the work-related themes expressed by lesbian parents in their interviews.

Instrumental Support

One theme central to relationships between lesbian parent households and mothers' work environments was the availability of instrumental support for the family of the worker. However, although most respondents mentioned salary and benefits when asked to describe supports and stressors in the household-work relationship, their comments emphasized that money was not the only motivation for their work. This view of work as "more than a paycheck" is in keeping with an earlier study of heterosexual mothers whose views reflected their realization that work co-existed with individual and family needs (Harold, Colarossi & Mercier, 1997). Terry, a finance professional, put it this way:

> If I could get paid more money for doing something else . . . then I would do something else. But I like what I do. If it didn't require 40-45 hours a week, that would be even better. But if I didn't like it, I wouldn't be there.

Comments about compensation were often tied to other concerns, such as the schedule of the full-time worker, or the ways in which one partner's salary allowed the other partner to be more available to the children. Chandra echoed this theme in describing her partner's work:

> She's full time–she's eight to five–and she makes good money. That's part of the reason I got to go down to part time–because she had a job change and makes good money. She makes $18 an hour, and I make $8, so there's quite a difference. She's the primary breadwinner.

Employment benefits, such as health insurance, paid vacation, and sick leave, can account for up to 40% of the value of a full-time position. But changes in the American workplace mean that many employees no longer have access to these standard benefits, and perks like flexible work schedules and child care assistance are increasingly rare (Caputo, 2000; Fredriksen-Goldsen & Scharlach, 2001). Nonetheless, access to benefits remains critical to most parents. Non-salary benefits were of central importance to the lesbian parents interviewed for this study, and access to these benefits was complicated by the unique social and legal conditions of these families. For example, access to second-parent adoption can provide substantial protection for children and parents in some lesbian parent families. Children born into or adopted into families headed by same-sex partners often have only one legal parent. Second-parent (or co-parent) adoption is the legal process that provides these children with the legal, financial, and psychological security of having two parents. Second-parent adoption is not applicable to families in which two biological or legal parents already exist, but it is an important mechanism for ensuring that those with only one legal parent have access to the co-parent's workplace benefits (Committee on Pyschosocial Aspects of Child and Family Health, 2002). Only three of the 15 families represented in this study had completed second-parent adoptions, and none lived in a state that recognized same-sex civil marriage. Lack of access to these legal protections meant that most of the women interviewed faced roadblocks to basic workplace benefits for their families.

Health insurance for partners and partners' children was most often mentioned as a desired but unavailable form of instrumental support. For most of the families interviewed, lack of benefits for family members meant that one partner, and sometimes the children, bought health insurance independently or had no health coverage. In all families, health coverage was uneven, complex, and a source of some concern and resentment. Lynn described her partner's work:

> (Cara) has no benefits. That's (a) big negative. I can't carry her on mine, but I can carry (the baby), so (the baby) and I have full benefits. And Cara's . . . we have to pay for.

Similarly, Chandra, who worked 25 hours a week, had a partner whose full time job offered excellent benefits, but not for Chandra or the children. Thus, Chandra went without health coverage, while her children in a state-sponsored health program for low-income children.

Although many respondents described themselves as open about their sexual orientation at work, statements about benefits discrimination were often accompanied by references to the heterosexism of the work environment. Concerns about job security and problems in relationships with employers were issues for respondents who desired insurance coverage for partner or dependents. Kerry's description is typical. When asked to describe the supports and stressors of the work place, she replied simply: "The benefit package is a stressor. Lack of benefits for my partner. (And) there's always the threat of . . . not spoken threat of . . . being discriminated against at work because of orientation."

The only one of the respondents ever to have had access to domestic partner benefits in the work place was Carolyn, whose former employer was a pioneer in offering health insurance and other benefits to same sex partners. Carolyn laughed when the interviewer asked if she had taken advantage of the domestic partner benefits in that job. Her description of her experience with that employer contradicts its image as a supportive, liberal environment:

> I couldn't get out of there fast enough. Well it was a great job, but a combination of dysfunctional work place, anti-gay, right wing creeps. . . . You know, I was adopting children and I was scared to tell anyone because I was afraid someone would stop it because I was (lesbian) . . . (There were) some real anti-gay people there. The most wonderful experience of my life (adopting the girls) and I was scared to death, you know?

In addition to comments about salary and health insurance, respondents mentioned the value of job stability and security as forms of instrumental support in the work place. These factors were particularly important to the 9 families in which income from one partner supported the rest of the family.

Interpersonal Support

A second central theme of the respondents' descriptions of household-work relationships was the availability of interpersonal support in the work place environment. While none of the interviewees made interpersonal relationships primary to descriptions of their interactions with work, nevertheless most mentioned co-workers at some time in the interviews. Nearly all respondents reported being out as lesbians at work, and most described interpersonal relationships that had a positive impact on the household-work interaction. Chandra, who works in an elementary school, described the person-to-person interaction as a highlight of her job:

> (The relationship type's) gotta be strong positive because I get along with everybody there. There's the pay, yeah, but what're you going to do? It's the one negative. It's actually a dream job, and I like working with the kids too–they crack me up. What job do you have that, when you walk in, everybody jumps up and hugs you? Everybody's happy to see you and they run down to me. You don't walk into the office (in most jobs) and have people do that . . .

In a few cases, the value of adult interaction on the job was most evident in comments from and about women who were stay-at-home mothers. That is, interpersonal support as a benefit of employment was most evident in its absence. Julie described her reaction to staying home with her son:

> This is really the first time that I haven't been working. And you get a lot of your self-esteem from working. So even though I am working, it's just not the same as working out in the public. You know, even though I get a lot of kudos for how well (my child) is doing, (it's not the same).

In addition to comments on the benefits of interpersonal relationships at work, a few respondents mentioned less-positive interactions with co-workers and supervisors. Chandra mentioned that her partner's conflict with her supervisor could threaten her job security. Similarly, Bonnie, an attorney with a fairly prestigious job, commented that she felt little control in her relationship with her supervisor: And several women reported that anti-lesbian sentiment created noxious work environments. Candace mentioned that her partner has had some interruption in co-worker relationships since coming out as lesbian:

> She has received some grief from people. Just a lot of her closer friends let her go at work . . . And then I think (it was) probably me . . . being with a woman. I think that they (thought) 'How could she give up a man for a woman?'

Marla, too, reported that attitudes toward lesbian and gay issues in the work place have impacted her partner's interpersonal experiences at work:

> This work environment is so much better for her than her last work environment, where there was a principal who, just right in front of the whole school, was cutting down gays and everything. It was just the most awful environment. She was the only, that she *knew of*, gay person on the staff. Now, this is a much different working environment. She has open gay staff members and it feels much more supportive.

In Tamara's case, the interaction with her co-workers was a combination of support as a lesbian and frustration with her status as parent. Tamara described her relationships in an agency with a high percentage of gay and lesbian employees:

> In general, compared to a lot of jobs, it's been a really strong, supportive relationship. Well, part of it (is) just being able to be real out here. And you know, people knowing how much I wanted to have kids, and to be supportive of that.

As these statements suggest, the issue of interpersonal support in the work place was quite complex. Personality, work place culture and policies, job type and setting all interacted with respondents' styles of communication, degree of openness, and myriad other factors with various outcomes.

Integration of Work and Family

Another major theme of household-work relationships was how workplace supports allowed respondents to be available for their children. This issue was of preeminent concern for most parents. For lesbian parent families, the integration of work and family was the theme expressed most often by the women interviewed, and the complexity of their needs was well-articulated.

One way that respondents measured the potential integration of work and family was in the flexibility offered by the work place. Allowance for variations in scheduled work hours, and schedules that paralleled school and day care were considered valuable perks to these mothers. For example, when explaining her decision to leave behind her former job's salary, benefits and security, Carolyn said:

> No schedule fits when you have kids. I don't care what it is. You know, you get a schedule, and then their naps change or their day care changes because they get older. And then that doesn't work any more. I didn't want to have to be somewhere (away from the kids).

Just as flexibility was noted as a benefit, any lack of availability for children's activities, appointments and other events was seen as a particular hardship by these parents. Even workers with positions that seemed to promise a high degree of independence mentioned the desire to be more available for their children. Julie commented on their 'special-needs' son's weekly medical and therapy appointments, which her partner is unable to attend:

> It's hard when there's things going on that she should be a part of that she can't be a part of. I mean, she makes it to all of his major appointments, but you almost kind of feel resentful that she can't be there for, like, the therapy appointments and things like that. Just so she can see first-hand what's going on with him.

Another way that respondents measured the intersection of work and family life was by co-workers' and bosses' expressions of acceptance of children. Generally, familiarity with the needs of children and families, whether by formal policy or informal interaction, was considered an asset in the work place. Thus, several respondents mentioned that allowing partners and children to call the work place, including partners and children in work-related social activities, and other related behaviors contributed to positive household-work relationships.

A few families experienced work as an agent separating the employee from partner and children. Kerry described how her partner's supervisor required her partner to attend classes that take her away from the family nearly every evening of the week. Jocelyn complained that her partner's work hours were a serious impediment to their time together. Julie described trying to call her partner on the telephone:

> I always feel bad when I have to call (Joan) at work, because I'm afraid that she's gonna get in trouble. And so it's stressful for me when I have to call her. And if she has to take a day off, I'm always worried that she's gonna make somebody mad or get on somebody's list. And it seems like, just recently, she's had to take more time off than normal because there's things going on (with our son).

Simple access to family members who were out of the home all day was a frequently-mentioned issue. Workplace policies that prohibited or discouraged family communication were attributed to employers who were "business-minded" or otherwise inhumane. In contrast, family-friendly practices in the work place were often credited to administrators who were parents, or who liked children. Julie continued:

> Joan's just transferred jobs within the same company. The supervisor that she had before was very supportive. He told her, 'If you need off, don't worry about it. Take it.' The supervisor that she has now has no children, and has no real understanding of, you know, when your child is sick or needs to go to the cardiologist.

Similarly, work-related social activities that included partners and children were mentioned as a support for families. Several respondents said that their partners were "invited" to staff parties and comparable events, but some described a workplace culture that excluded the children. Tamara described her childless co-workers' decision to exclude her children from an activity:

> I'll give you an example. I thought this was real funny. Our staff said, 'Let's plan a trip to (an amusement park) or something.' And basically folks just said, 'Okay, we're all going to go, but just take partners, not kids.' Can you imagine saying to your kids: 'I'm sorry, I'm taking the day off, going to (the amusement park) with my grown-up friends and you can't go?' So, it's like, 'Have fun, you guys!'

Descriptions of work schedules, opportunities for time away from work to attend to family business, and inclusion of partners and children in work-related social activities reflected respondents' desire to reconcile the need to work with the responsibilities of parenting and family life. Those with employment that allowed for integration of the two spheres invariably characterized their jobs as sources of support for their families. Interestingly, the three respondents who characterized household-work relationships as 'stressful / negative' on the interview eco maps identified lack of integration between work and family as primary stressors. These three families shared a number of characteristics: in each, the oldest child was a pre-schooler, only one partner worked full-time, the work place was a social service agency, and complaints centered on dislike for the stressful work or unpleasant co-workers. Respondents' descriptions in all three cases suggested that a combination of stressful work and noxious work environment led to a lack of home-work integration, and thus contributed to poor household-work relationships.

Strategies for Balancing Work and Family

As the data on integrating work and family indicate, an important focus for the respondents was the stress that they experienced in their dual roles as mothers and providers. Working parents manage the conflict between work and family in various ways. When a working parent can choose which of a variety of competing responsibilities will get priority, she expends energy to coordinate the various roles. The effort needed in this coordination is termed role strain (Warren & Johnson, 1995). But when role demands occur simultaneously and none can be deferred, as when a child's medical appointment conflicts with an important business meeting, some parents attempt to deal with the conflict by redefining roles and responsibilities within and outside of the family. Women who work outside the home commonly experience guilt about not being fully available to their families, and many use the strategy of 'role expansion' to deal these demands (Gilbert, Holahan & Manning,1981). That is, they add new responsibilities to their existing work-loads, without deleting existing tasks, in an attempt to do it all (Yogev, 1981). Often, these competing demands from work and family, termed 'interrole conflict,' are associated with feelings of dissatisfaction, less-effective parenting, and problems in job performance (Kossek & Ozeki, 1998). Bonnie described the problem:

> See, I feel like the ability to concentrate (at work) is way down be-
> cause I know I gotta do the dishwasher, and the laundry, and I just
> have to keep going. And I have to fill up the car with gas on Friday
> and on Sunday and, you know, it's so much (that) it's hard to con-
> centrate well.

The mainstream social science literature suggests that many women respond to parenthood by reducing their emphasis on employment (e.g. Bielby & Bielby, 1989). This study illustrated the variety of strategies used by respondents and their partners to manage the stress of balancing work and home life. Many families chose to give up the benefits of two full time incomes in favor of greater flexibility and availability to children. Others located full time positions that offered greater freedom to schedule their work hours around their children's needs. A few families, especially those with older children, managed to maintain full-time work with little interruption.

A small portion of the sample reported keeping personal and family spheres as separate as possible. The disconnection between work and home occurred only in families in which the worker was a step-parent in the household. In these cases, a step-parent is a woman who formed a new family by partnering with a woman and her children from a previous relationship or adoption. Beyond that commonality, the separation seemed to be unique in each of the families. Chandra's partner was described as a person who "just doesn't talk about things (including her family)" in her corporate job. Candace described her part time work in an office where she is the only female employee: "Well, I've not really told anyone (that I'm lesbian). I work with all men . . . keep my personal life, my personal life and my work life, my work life."

Terry's position about dissociating personal and professional roles was the most strongly stated. She explained why she does not pursue interpersonal relationships at work beyond those required to get her job done:

> For me, since I'm a manager at work, my whole philosophy since I
> started working, is that I've seen too many women, in particular,
> where no matter how supportive companies are, they tend to pick
> on personal issues for women. So what I do is, I do my job. I do it
> well. You know, I advance through my career but I don't bring the
> personal side into it, because I don't want that to be an influence.
> I've seen it happen too many times, with women in particular.

Terry's depiction of the work place as a place to "do my job (and) do it well" was not common in this sample. In truth, there was a remarkable lack of focus on ambition, professional accomplishment, or the details of careers, considering the level of education and expertise in the group of interviewees. More frequently, respondents reported on ways that they worked to balance work and family without separating the two completely. In addition to choosing employment that allowed for increased flexibility in work hours, several respondents mentioned strategies for *limiting* the impact of work life in the home. Jocelyn, for example described her family's simple strategy for controlling the impact of her partner's work on the family:

> (My partner) works 12 hour days, five days a week. Usually, no less than 12 hours. Sometimes 14! Her schedule's always changing. She's stressed. Sometimes, you know, she brings home work, like we all do, and she's stressed about it for a while. And she gets a lot of calls, you know, she tends to get calls at home. Sometimes they're late night calls because the restaurant closes . . . sometimes they're closing till 12 or 1 a.m. So we've got calls at midnight before. Now, we just don't answer (the phone). We just don't answer it.

Another, more common, strategy mentioned by respondents combined worker efficiency with work place flexibility. This approach often resulted in *increased* interaction between work place and home life, with the worker asserting control and independence in the relationship. Amy reported flexing her schedule without consulting with anyone so that she can provide transportation, after-school care and other needs. Lynn takes her infant to work with her nearly every day, sometimes even asking her supervisor to care for the child when she has to attend to business that cannot include the baby.

In all, respondents described a wide variety of pragmatic and creative strategies for managing work and family. Throughout their interviews, these women were clear that family is important to them, and thus worth the stress and compromise of juggling dual roles. Respondents were quite optimistic about their ability to manage their work lives to maximize their effectiveness as parents. The comments of Marla, who runs a child care business in her home, reflect the sentiments of many of the mothers interviewed:

> At first I was a little jealous of the time that the other kids took away from my own kids. The reason I was doing this (child care

business) was that I wanted to be home with my own kids. It was me learning to put my own priorities . . . that my own kids come first. These are my clients and my charges and they're very important too, but . . . I've learned how to work that out and to balance it.

DISCUSSION

The data on household-work relationships revealed that lesbian parents attend to both the instrumental and interpersonal aspects of employment. Benefits like salary, health insurance, and job security are highly valued. In the same way, personal support, friendly interactions, and the inclusion of partners and children in the social aspects of the work culture are important. The need to be both parent and worker was a source of stress for most of the women interviewed. A few women coped with the pressure of the home-family interaction by separating the spheres, but, as their work profiles indicate, many of these women demonstrated willingness to take risks and to use creativity in the workplace by balancing pay and perks with flexibility in work schedules.

Analysis of the data on relationships between lesbian parent families and mothers' work yielded several important themes. The women interviewed for this study were remarkably open about sexual orientation in their jobs. Most respondents enjoyed positive interpersonal relationships with supervisors and coworkers, although a few women reported that disclosure of sexual orientation had negative consequences for their work relationships. Research in the 1980's indicated that the majority of lesbians feared losing their jobs if their sexual orientation were revealed to their employers (Levine & Leonard, 1984; Poverny & Finch, 1988). Although overt discrimination does not seem to be a *primary* concern for most, these data suggest that some lesbian parents continue to deal with stigma in the workplace.

As might be expected in a sample with this level of commitment to family, most of the respondents described family work arrangements that allowed at least one parent to spend substantial time with her child or children. Entrepreneurship, part time jobs, use of flexible schedules, and choosing to live on a single income were strategies used by respondents in this study. These and other approaches to balancing work and family support the notion that lesbian parents are creative and adaptable in their relationships with work, often placing accessibility to children above benefits, job security and salary.

The focus on integration of work and family can be seen as evidence of lesbian parents' commitment to maintaining the integrity of their families (Lott-Whitehead & Tully, 1993). Comments about the value placed on the inclusion of partners and children in work-related social events support this interpretation, as do data on the negative impact of inflexibility in workers' schedules. Gender socialization doubtless provides a parallel explanation for this finding. That is, families with two mothers may be likely to make decisions that favor interpersonal relationships and children's needs over financial achievement because women are socialized to value nurturing of partners and children above all other concerns. More research is needed to clarify this issue, and to examine the ways in which lesbian parents make decisions about the work-family balance at various stages of family and child development.

The issue of health care benefits for partners and children was one area of the household-work relationship for which respondents were unable to devise creative solutions. Nearly all the women interviewed accepted lack of access to health insurance for family members as a fact of modern American life. Although some respondents mentioned the desire for domestic partner policies as a way to access benefits, most seemed to consider change in their benefits impossible.

Implications for Policy Practice

Lesbian parent families exist outside of the mainstream of public life in many important ways. Attention must be given to policies that support members of these families as legitimate, contributing, responsible workers, community members and citizens. Respondents in this study reported on the everyday realities of their lives, and their comments were based on their experiences and beliefs rather than their ambitions. For this reason, perhaps, none of the women interviewed mentioned same-sex marriage as a potential solution to concerns in the workplace. For them, a more immediate and attainable solution may lie with progressive workplace family policies that directly impact access to needed benefits. Increasing numbers of employers offer some form of domestic partner benefits. In 2006, more than half of Fortune 500 companies offered the benefits, and nearly all (92%) of the nation's top universities offered health coverage to gay and lesbian employees' families (Human Rights Campaign Foundation, 2006). Despite employers' concerns about the adverse fiscal impact of domestic partner policies, the effects are estimated to be small; employer costs would increase between 1.4% and 2.1% (Ash & Badgett, 2006).

As the data show, in reality one or both partners in a lesbian two-parent family may have difficulty accessing health insurance, disability, and retirement plans if they work at jobs that are less than full-time, stay at home to raise children, or choose to be self-employed. Even in families where a parent is a full-time worker who enjoys excellent benefits, children may not have health insurance and other coverage if the worker is not the legal or biological parent of the children. Commitment to the family is socially desirable, and policies ought to support workers who take their parenting roles seriously. Greater availability of domestic partner benefits could create a safety net for lesbian parent families by ensuring that access to work place benefits does not come at the price of decreased availability for children's needs.

Women who are responsible for supporting their children ought to be identified as parents for the purposes of workplace and other social benefits. In this study, most respondents who had access to second-parent adoption used it. Like domestic partner benefits, women in this study seemed to see second-parent adoption as more realistic and more desirable than same-sex marriage. In addition, second-parent adoption focuses on the needs of the children, rather than on the partner relationship, so may better reflect the goals of these women while avoiding the religious and social implications of marriage.

Federal and state protections for lesbians and gay men, and smaller-scale policy changes for domestic partner benefits and second-parent adoption have long been the arena of gay and lesbian activists. Social workers and others who are mandated to work for social justice must join the struggle to achieve equity for lesbian parent families. To do otherwise is to ignore a fundamental civil rights issue and social service opportunity of our era.

Implications for Direct Practice

The sample of lesbian parent families used in this research had remarkably few problems that might merit the intervention of a psychiatric social worker, psychologist or physician. By virtue of their need for services, lesbian parent families in clinical populations are likely to exhibit a variety of problems not mentioned here, and many may need intensive intervention. This study did not aim to search out potential pathologies in lesbian parent families. Nevertheless, the results of this research suggest principles of intervention that are particularly salient with lesbian parents and their children.

Before working with lesbian parents, practitioners will benefit from increasing their understanding of the values, beliefs and behaviors that guide these mothers' interactions within the household and in the community. The sample of lesbians studied here, for example, displayed a remarkable commitment to their roles as parents, even at the expense of financial prosperity. In addition, interdependence was the rule in these families and is seen clearly in these data on family work arrangements. Of course, just as the women interviewed here expressed these themes in different ways, clients will vary in their presentation of issues that have most meaning for them. A thorough and directed assessment must include family work arrangements and related concerns, such as parental availability for children and access to work place benefits.

Once assessment is completed, planning for intervention should include consideration of clients' characteristic methods of approaching solution development. This study showed strong support for the notion that lesbian parents use creative and flexible approaches to problem solving. For example, some respondents reported that they solved the dilemma of managing work and family by moving from traditional jobs into self-employment. Examination of the methods by which parents' manage the work-family relationship may provide a template for further problem solving. Although this suggestion sounds simplistic, it may be quite difficult for some practitioners. While none of the parents in this study could be characterized as highly deviant, practitioners who value safety and conformity might experience solutions developed in this way as non-traditional, or even risky.

The results of this study clearly highlight intersections between individuals in lesbian parent families and institutions in the community as areas of particular strain. Understanding the meanings that members of families ascribe to instances of subtle bias or miscommunication is essential to effective intervention. Because much of the pressure experienced in household-community relationships amounts to institutionalized heterosexism, conscientious practitioners may need to act as advocates for their clients. In addition to advocacy, micro practice methods that empower lesbian parents to develop their own systems of support and intervention should be considered. For example, referral to support groups or on-line communities for lesbian parents would minimize the need for each family to discover the most effective ways of dealing with workplace pressures. Participation in support groups is also a way for lesbian parents and children to meet and develop friendships, thereby increasing overall social support.

Of course, in order for these referrals to be effective, practitioners need to increase awareness of community resources for lesbian parents. In urban centers and liberal suburban communities, these resources may include gay and lesbian centers and existing lesbian parent support groups, but since many lesbian parent families live outside of these areas, other sources of support should be considered as well. Welcoming religious communities, feminist women's organizations, Internet groups, and lesbian publications can all be effective referrals for ongoing support, although each must be researched by the practitioner before being recommended.

CONCLUSION

The relationships between lesbian parent families and their social environments are fairly complex, and the analyses done here only begin to reveal the experiences of this group of interviewees. Although limited in many ways, the results of this study support previous research on lesbian parents and their children, although some of the strengths, stressors and motivations of lesbian parent families in their work-family relationships have not been discussed in the literature before. The results of this study should lead to further consideration of the particular strengths and coping strategies evident in members of other non-traditional families. Continued evaluation of such families is needed so that social service providers can better understand the ways in which marginalized communities are able to be successful. Without such understanding, further research and attempted intervention may grow increasingly irrelevant.

REFERENCES

Bielby, W. T., & Bielby, D. D. (1989). Family ties: Balancing commitments to work and family in dual earner households. *American Sociological Review, 54*, 776-789.

Cahill, S., Ellen, M. & Tobias, S. (2003). *Family policy: Issues affecting gay, lesbian, transgender and bisexual families.* Washington, D.C.: Policy Institute of the National Gay and Lesbian Task Force.

Caputo, R. K. (2000). The availability of traditional and family friendly benefits among a cohort of young women, 1968-95. *Families in Society, 81 (4)*, 422-436.

Committee on Pyschosocial Aspects of Child and Family Health. (2002). Coparent or second-parent adoption by same-sex parents. *Pediatrics, 109*, (2). 339-340.

Demo, D. & Allen, K. (1996). Diversity within lesbian and gay families: Challenges and implications for family theory and research. *Journal of Social and Personal Relations, 13* (3), 415-434.

Fonow, M., & Cook, J. (1991). Back to the future: A look at the second wave of feminist epistemology and methodology. In M. Fonow and J. Cook, (Eds.), *Beyond methodology: Feminist scholarship as lived research,* (pp. 1-15). Indianapolis, IN: Indiana University Press.

Fredriksen-Goldsen, K. I., & Scharlach, A. E. (2001). *Familes and work: New directions in the twenty-first century.* New York: Oxford University Press.

Gilbert, L. A., Holahan, C. K., & Manning, L. (1981). Coping with conflict between professional and maternal roles. *Family Relations, 30* (3), 419-426.

Gornick, J. C., & Meyers, M. K. (2001). Support for working families: What the United States can learn from Europe. *American Prospect, 12* (1), 3-7.

Harold, R. D., Colarossi, L. G., & Mercier, L. R. (2007). *Smooth sailing or stormy waters? Family transitions through adolescence and their implications for practice, policy and research.* Medwah, NJ: Lawrence Erlbaum Associates, Inc.

Harold, R. D., Mercier, L. R., & Colarossi, L. G. (1997). Using the eco-map to bridge the practice-research gap. *Journal of Sociology and Social Welfare, 24,* 29-44.

Harvard Law Review. (1990). *Sexual orientation and the law*: Cambridge. MA: Harvard University Press.

Human Rights Campaign Foundation. (2006). *The state of the workplace for gay, lesbian, bisexual and transgender Americans, 2005-2006.* Washington, D.C.: Human Rights Campaign Foundation.

Klerman, J. A., & Leibowitz, A. (1990). Child care and women's return to work after child-birth. *American Economic Review, 80,* 284-288.

Kossek, E. E., & Ozeki, C. (1998). Work-family conflict, policies, and the job-life satisfaction relationship: A review and directions for organizational behavior-human resources research. *Journal of Applied Psychology, 83,* 139-149.

Laird, J. (1994). Lesbian families: A cultural perspective. *Smith College Studies in Social WorkI, 64 (3), 263-296.*

Levine, M. & Leonard, R. (1984). Discrimination against lesbians in the work force. *Signs, 9* (4), 700-710.

Lott-Whitehead, L & Tully, C. (1993). The family lives of lesbian mothers. *Smith College Studies in Social Work, 63* (3), 265-280.

McDonald, H. B. & Steinhorn, A. I. (1993). *Understanding homosexuality: A guide for those who know, love or counsel gay and lesbian individuals.* New York: Crossroad.

Mercier, L. R., & Harold, R. D. (2001). Job talk: The role of work in family life. In R. D. Harold (Ed.), *Becoming a family: Parents stories and their implications for practice, policy and research (pp. 155-193).* Mahwah, New Jersey: Lawrence Erlbaum Associates.

Parks, C. (1998). Lesbian parenthood: A review of the literature. *American Journal of Orthopsychiatry,* 68 (3), 376-389.

Parsons, T. & Bales, R. (1955). *Family, socialization and interaction process.* New York: Free Press.

Poverny, L. M. & Finch, W. A. (1988). Gay and lesbian domestic partnerships: Expanding the definition of family. *Social Casework, 69,* 116-121.

Singleton, J. (2000). Women caring for elderly family members: Shaping non-traditional work and family initiatives. *Journal of Comparative Family Studies, 31* (3), 367

Smith, P. J., & Beaujot, R. (1999). Men's orientation toward marriage and family roles, *Journal of Comparative Family Studies,* 30 (3), 471-488.

Strauss, A. L., & Corbin, J. M. (1990). *Basics of qualitative research: grounded theory procedures and techniques.* Newbury Park, CA: Sage Publications.

Tully, C. T. (1995). *Lesbian social services: Research issues.* New York: Harrington Park Press.

Voydanoff, P. (1987). *Work and family life.* Newbury Park, CA: Sage.

Warren, J. A., & Johnson, P. J. (1995). The impact of workplace support on work-family role strain. *Family Relations,* 44 (2), 163-169.

Yogev, S. (1981). Do professional women have egalitarian marital relationships? *Journal of Marriage and the Family, 43* (4), 865-871.

A Model for Policy Analysis Applied to the *Goodridge* Case

Misty L. Wall

Marriage is one of the most basic civil rights of humans (Zablocki v Redhail, 1978). The institution of civil marriage aims to promote healthy families, to protect the economic, and emotional interdependence of family members, and to give priority to their bonds. Until November of 2003, same sex couples were excluded from the rights and responsibilities of marriage in every state in the United States. Legal protection of partner relationships increases a couple's ability to care for each other, offers access to more than 1,000 federally protected rights, and provides families security and peace of mind.

Marriage has evolved drastically over the past 200 years, and each change has been met with opposition from conservative interest groups, dating back to 1750, when it was declared "immoral" and "unnatural" to marry someone outside your own race. This law, now seen as a blatant act of oppression, inequality, and racism, did not come off the books until 1967 when the Supreme Court ruled in *Loving v. Virginia* (1967) that the ban on interracial marriage was a violation of the United States Constitution. Since that time, the institution of marriage has remained a controversial topic. Religious conservatives have pushed constitutional amendments that redefine marriage to exclude gay and lesbian couples. For example, the federal Defense of Marriage Act, or DOMA, is one of the largest efforts to limit the rights of same sex couples. DOMA redefines marriage to include "one man and one woman," therein denying gay and lesbian couples the more than 1000 benefits of federally recognized marriages.

The landmark ruling handed down in *Goodridge v. Department of Public Health* (2003) marked a highpoint in the struggle for equal rights for gay and lesbian individuals and couples. The justices who ruled in the *Goodridge (2003)* case recognized the significant civil liberties surrounding marriage, the importance of equality to all citizens, and the psychological and sociological importance of marriage. The goal of this paper is to analyze the recent judicial ruling in the *Goodridge* (2003) case in which the Supreme Court of Massachusetts granted same sex couples the right to legally recognized marriages within Massachusetts using a newly developed policy analysis model. The policy analysis model is designed to provide a method to understand the legal, political, and value driven issues surrounding a judicial decision.

THE MODEL

The policy analysis model applied within this paper is a logical six-step process designed by the author to be used during analysis of judicial decisions. The process begins with establishing the circumstances that led to a request for legal intervention. The second step is to identify the issues involved in the case; the analysis must determine what each party (the plaintiff and defendant) is asking the court to grant. Once the requests are clearly identified, the analyst must consider what arguments are presented in support of each party's request. The third step is a logical progression of the second. In step two, supporting and opposing arguments were identified. The third step calls for evaluation of each party's argument. In this context, evaluation consists of using literature and outcome data to determine the validity of each side's arguments.

The fourth step in the model is the application of Moroney's (1981) value criteria. One way that societal values are expressed is through law and court decisions. There are times that court decisions are directly in line with the majority of citizens. Likewise, there are times that the vision of the court to extend and preserve civil rights has been ahead of the majority. For instance, the Supreme Court ruling to end school segregation was vehemently opposed by most US citizens. In fact, the very idea of a social issue implies an unrealized social value (Iatridis, 1994). Thus, value criteria are at the heart of all social policy (Moroney, 1981) and clearly apparent in the *Goodridge (2003)* case. Including value criteria in the model forces the analysis to formally acknowledge the value(s) at the heart of the policy issues identified and the role they play in the judicial decision and analysis. In step four, the policy analyst should consider the role of values in each party's argument, which values are maximized, and which are minimized by the judicial ruling.

Next, the analyst should complete an interest analysis. Interest analysis identifies those people or groups who are affected, directly, indirectly, or not at all by the ruling. Many times a court decision affects many more people than intended and may take many years for the effects to be fully recognized. None the less, the court decision was made in an effort to impact someone or something, and those affected must be anticipated and assessed in order for an analysis to be effective and accurate. Interest analysis also aims to anticipate ways that each group of individuals may respond.

Step six is a logical progression from interest analysis, as it builds on the anticipated responses of groups of individuals. In step six, the policy analysis considers alternative remedies that would meet the needs of people involved. Exploring alternatives is a common step in many policy analysis models. However, it has not been applied to the few models designed to address judicial decisions. Policy analysts strive to understand a policy, in this case a court decision. In understanding such a topic one must look at all the possible aspects of achieving the desired outcome. A judicial decision, especially at the Supreme Court level, is a reflection of an evolutionary process and to skip consideration of alternative makes analysis a static process, well outside of the spirit of the legal process.

APPLICATION OF THE MODEL TO GOODRIDGE V. DEPARTMENT OF PUBLIC HEALTH *(2003)*

Step One: Establishing the Facts

During March and April of 2001, seven same sex couples applied for marriage licenses in various counties in Massachusetts. The Department of Public Health, the body that is responsible for issuing marriage licenses, denied the couples' requests. The reason the requests were denied is that all of the couples applied to marry their same sex partner. Subsequently the couples field a lawsuit against the Department of Public Health. GLAD (Gay and Lesbian Advocates and Defenders) represented all seven couples until the final ruling was issued on November 11, 2003.

By a four to three margin, the Supreme Court of Massachusetts invalidated the exclusion of same sex couples from marriage. The court reformulated the common law definition of civil marriage to "the voluntary union of two persons as spouses, to the exclusion of all others." This was a landmark ruling in favor of the seven couples represented in *Goodridge v. Department of Public Heath* (2003), as well as gay and lesbian rights. The court's decision recognized the cultural, financial, and political importance of marriage to all citizens, regardless of sexual orientation.

Step Two: Identifying the Policy Issues

One model of judicial analysis, developed by Turnbull (1981), suggests that it is helpful to re-examine and restate the policies that are reflected in the state's statute and the relationships of family members with each other and the government. Stated another way, through re-examination of policies we are able to clearly articulate what each party is asking the court to grant.

In the *Goodridge* (2003) case, the Plaintiffs' arguments were centered around the wording in the Massachusetts Constitution, which demands equitable treatment and liberty for all citizens, forbids the creation of second-class citizens, and affords all citizens due process. The Plaintiffs argued they were denied all these rights when the Department of Public Health denied their requests for marriage licenses.

The Defendant in the *Goodridge* (2003) case, the Department of Public Health, argued that the Constitution did not extend to gay couples because the intent of the Constitution was to advance marriage for the primary reason of procreation. They also contended that heterosexual marriage, consisting of two parents, one of each sex, created the optimal setting to raise children. The third argument presented by the defense was that denying same sex couples the right to marry served the state by preservation of scarce financial resources (*Goodridge v. Department of Public Heath*, 2003).

By identifying what each party hoped to gain (what they are asking the court to grant) the true policy issues become evident. At first glance, the issue central in the *Goodridge (2003)* case may appear to be the seven denied marriage licenses. However, further exploration reveals the deeper political issue. The issue in *Goodridge v. Department of Public Health* (2003) is one of equally (or unequally) distributed civil liberty. A civil liberty is a guaranteed right which is beyond the power of government to restrict. Civil liberties commonly exercised by Americans include freedom of religion, freedom to marry, freedom to have a family, and freedom from torture.

Step Three: Evaluation of Supporting/Opposing Arguments

Evaluation of supporting and opposing arguments begins with understanding the legal basis for each argument. In order for an argument to be entertained by the court, it must be originated from an established or emerging right. An established right is one that has been deemed inalienable by the Constitution. An emerging right, which the rights of gay and lesbian persons are considered to be, is less concrete. Establishing a right in the eyes of the court occurs by hearing cases in which groups of people have stated that they feel they have been excluded from certain liberties. The *Goodridge* (2003) case explores the right to civil marriage.

The central question in the *Goodridge* (2003) case is one of constitutional rights. The arguments presented by the Plaintiff's in the *Goodridge (2003)* case were possible because the Massachusetts Constitution specifically calls for equality and liberty to all citizens, it forbids making any citizen a second-class citizen, and guarantees each citizen due process in the face of dissention.

Once a new right, or clarification of a right, is determined to be appropriate, the court must decide how to impose the changes. In the case of *Goodridge v. Department of Public Health* (2003), the court amended the Massachusetts Constitution, changing the definition of marriage to clearly extend to all citizens, regardless of sexual orientation.

The arguments presented by the Department of Public Health in the *Goodridge* (2003) case were also based on an interpretation of the Massachusetts Constitution. The Plaintiffs interpreted the omission of wording in the Constitution that clearly excluded same sex marriage as an indication that same sex marriage is in keeping with the spirit of the state's constitution. Meanwhile, the Department of Public Health argued the original intent of marriage, as protected in the Massachusetts Constitution, is procreation. They argued that because same sex couples are unable to biologically conceive their partner's child, they are not intended to be protected under the state's constitution. The court considered this argument, but ultimately dismissed it stating there was no logical, or legal, connection between fertility and the institution of marriage. The court further stated that this defense failed to consider heterosexual couples who marry without the intention of having children, as well as those heterosexual couples unable to biologically conceive their spouse's child.

The Department's second argument was that homosexual parenting is not an acceptable situation in which to raise children. Considerable qualitative and quantitative research has been conducted with gay and lesbian parents and their children. To date all valid research shows that gay and lesbian parents are equally capable of raising children and that children raised by gay and lesbian parents are not hindered psychologically, psychosocially, or cognitively (Flaks, Ficher, Masterpasqua, & Joseph, 1995; Falk, 1989, Green, Mandel, Hotvedt, Gray, & Smith, 1986; Golombock, Spencer, & Rutter, 1983, Harris & Turner 1985, Huggins, 1989; Kirkpatrick, Smith & Roy, 1981; Gottman, 2001).

The third argument presented by the Department concerned the preservation of scarce state financial resources. The Department argued that the state had a compelling reason to deny same sex couples the right to marry, because the more people who are married, the more benefits the government has to provide. The Department also argued that same sex couples are less dependent on each other financially than are heterosexual married couples. They based this argument on the assumption that same sex couples have not been able to share debt in the ways that heterosexual couples traditionally have. The court found this to be inconsistent with the facts presented in the *Goodridge* (2003) case, as several of the Plaintiffs have children, and two of the Plaintiffs are mutually caring for elderly parents. The court also stated that heterosexual couples do not have to prove they are financially reliant on each other to receive state supported assistance, only that they are married. The court concluded that there was no reasonable correlation between denying same sex couples the right to marry and the state's economy. In fact, outcome data for areas that have approved same sex civil unions indicate an increase in revenue via tourism (Sailer, 2003).

Although the Department did not directly argue that homosexuality is immoral, the court received a number of amicus briefs on behalf of groups that felt this way. The court responded to these arguments in the summary. The court pointed out that at the time of the *Goodridge* (2003) ruling, 59% of Massachusetts residents favored same sex couples being granted the right to marry (*Goodridge v. Department of Public Health*, 2003) and even more believed that same sex couples should have more rights than they currently had. The court also pointed to prior litigation within the state, including decriminalization of sodomy, expanding partnership benefits, custody and visitation being granted to gay and lesbian parents, and state code's protecting gay men and lesbians from discrimination by state agencies. The court deemed these actions, which were all supported by Massachusetts citizens, to be evidence of a growing tolerance for same sex couples.

Step Four: Value Criteria

In the *Goodridge* (2003) case, the policy issues are heavily laden with moral values. The core issues can be compared to Moroney's (1981) value criteria of liberty, equity/equality, and fraternity. Moroney (1981) assumes three basic value criteria are the driving forces of all social policy. Moroney (1981) also assumes the position that not all values can be maximized simultaneously. Rather, each issue maximizes and minimizes each value criteria. It is the position of this author that the values of liberty, equality/equity, and fraternity are all increased by the *Goodridge* (2003) decision.

The value of liberty concerns choices, freedom, and options. The *Goodridge* (2003) ruling maximizes liberty by offering same sex couples the freedom, choice, and option to marry if they desire. Equality is maximized by the *Goodridge* (2003) ruling, in that same sex couples were given the same opportunity to marry, to access services, and to the benefits and responsibilities of civil marriage. The *Goodridge* (2003) ruling also requires that Massachusetts counties fairly distribute marriage licenses to same sex couples.

From the perspective of same sex couples, fraternity is also maximized. Courts have a history of recognizing the importance of marriage in relation to community, well being, safety, and unity. The *Goodridge* (2003) ruling maximizes fraternity by granting same sex couples access to these same benefits. From the perspective of those in opposition to the ruling, fraternity is minimized because the ruling is not in conjunction, and thus threatens, their ideas of morality, unity, community, and safety.

Step Five: Interest Analysis

People who will be directly and indirectly affected by the court decision must be identified in the process of policy analysis. Turnbull (1981) refers to this process as interest analysis. According to Turnbull (1981), interest analysis is a technique used to dissect everyone's stakes in the case and possible outcomes. A modified version of Turnbull's (1981) interest analysis is utilized in this model. Interest analysis will be achieved by asking the following series of five questions.

Who is directly affected by the case?

Most obviously, the seven couples represented in *Goodridge* (2003) are affected by the ruling, because they can now be married within their state. Additionally, all gay and lesbian couples who are residents of Massachusetts, and who wish to be married, are also affected directly by the *Goodridge* (2003) ruling, because they now have the freedom to legally marry in that state. The children of the Plaintiffs in *Goodrigde* (2003) are also directly affected because they immediately gain the extra protection of having two legal parents. Finally, the state of Massachusetts is affected because its processes will have to be amended to include same sex couples.

Who is affected indirectly by the case?

In policy analysis it is important to evaluate the effectiveness of legislation through quantification. Although all gay men and lesbian women who wish to be married are undoubtedly directly affected by the Goodridge ruling, it is difficult to quantify the number of men and women this includes. Many gay men and lesbian women remain unwilling to identify their sexual orientation for fear of retaliation, making it difficult to gain an accurate estimate of how many people are directly affected by the ruling. One way to estimate the number is to use government data; the 2000 Census surveyed 105.5 million households, of which 4.9 million were heterosexual married couples, and 594,000 had partners of the same sex (U.S. Census Bureau, 2000).

Since the 2003 *Goodridge* ruling, many gay and lesbian couples have entered Massachusetts with the sole desire to be married. Subsequently, access to same sex marriage has been limited by rulings of the Massachusetts Supreme Court. In September 2006, the Massachusetts Supreme Court upheld a 1913 state law that limits civil marriage in Massachusetts to residents of Massachusetts or neighboring Rhode Island (Gay and Lesbian Advocates and Defenders, 2007). Others states are also indirectly affected as similar cases are likely to be heard in Supreme Courts in every state in the country. Also, as we have seen in the conservative firestorm following the *Goodridge* (2003) decision, many states are scrambling to amend their constitution before judges have an opportunity to rule in favor of same sex marriage in their state.

In addition, religious and antigay groups, who have actively opposed same sex marriage, are affected by the *Goodridge* (2003) ruling. Children of other gay and lesbian couples who wish to marry are also affected directly by the verdict.

Who is not affected by the case?

The *Goodridge* (2003) ruling does not influence the various religions or churches. Each faith may still choose which unions to officiate and recognize. Additionally, other states in the United Stated are currently under no obligation to recognized same sex marriages granted in Massachusetts.

What is each affected person or group likely to do?

Some same sex couples are likely to marry and begin utilizing the rights, responsibilities, and privileges associated with that union. Religious conservative groups are likely to strengthen their fight to redefine marriage through discriminatory legislation such as DOMA and Resolution 56. Resolution 56 would amend the US Constitution to define marriage to the union of a man and a woman and prevent legislators or courts from mandating more limited benefits such as civil unions and partnerships (Cahill & Slater, 2004).

Step Six: Consider Alternative Remedies

The alternatives to legally sanctioned marriage for gay and lesbian couples most commonly discussed are civil unions and domestic partnerships. When comparing marriage alternatives three primary factors should be considered.

Both local and federal governments provide benefits to married couples; these benefits must be assessed during policy analysis. Opinions in the US have gradually been expanding to provide legal protection and benefits to LGBT individuals. Twenty two states now include sexual orientation in their hate crime legislation (http://www.thetaskforce.org/reports_and_research/hate_crimes_laws), indicating a growing tolerance of gay men and lesbian women and a national commitment to equally protect all citizens. And although there appears to be a growing tolerance, extending equal rights to gay men and lesbians continue to be met with fierce resistance, thus understanding the benefits of civil marriage and marriage alternatives is a critical step in judicial analysis. Civil unions became popular in the United States in 2000 when the Vermont Supreme Court ruled in *Maker v. Vermont* (2000) that the state should grant same sex couples the same rights and privileges under Vermont law. Opposition to same sex marriage grew nationally and Vermont decided to create a separate institution designed recognize same sex couples relationships. Vermont lawmakers did this to comply with the Vermont Supreme Court mandate, but also to preserve the right of true civil marriage for heterosexual couples, thus solidifying civil marriage as an exclusive status unattainable to gay men and lesbians. Currently, versions of civil unions are available to gay and lesbian couples in Vermont, Connecticut, and New Jersey.

Since civil unions are recognized only at the state level, none of the federal benefits of marriage are extended. The ability to file joint taxes is another federally protected benefit of marriage not extended to those same sex couples who have had a civil union. Without the federal recognition of marriage, the benefits of civil unions or of a Massachusetts same sex marriage are gravely limited.

Portability, or stability of benefits when transported geographically, is also a critical limitation of civil unions. Currently, the only states in the United States granting civil unions are Vermont, Connecticut, and

New Jersey. This has implications for couples who are civil unionized because unions performed in these states will not be transported to any other state. For instance, if a couple has a legally registered same sex civil union and are visiting Texas on vacation, none of the rights or privileges provided by their civil union are recognized while outside the state.

The third consideration is the availability of civil unions. Availability in this situation refers to the locations that permit same sex unions. Traditional civil marriage is available across the globe. However, civil unions are currently only available inside the United States to residents of Vermont, Connecticut, and New Jersey. Internationally, more than that ten countries grant civil unions.

Another alternative to marriage is a registered domestic partnership. Domestic partnerships identify the personal relationship between individuals living together and sharing a common domestic life together. Currently each state decides on which benefits extended to registered domestic partners, and six states (California, District of Columbia, Hawaii, Maine, Maryland, and New York) offer some version of domestic partnerships. However, some private industries across the nation are providing some benefits to domestic partners such are insurance coverage for same sex couples.

Domestic partnerships generally allow same sex couples to register with the state to receive state supported benefits such as filing joint state income taxes, and in some cases, the ability to jointly adopt children, and guarantee hospital visitations. While the benefits of domestic partnerships can include all state supported benefits, no federal benefits are included.

As with civil unions, the portability of domestic partnerships is limited. No other state or locality has to recognize a registered domestic partnership or offer the same benefits the couple was previously receiving. Thus, regardless of how many states or localities adopt domestic partnership registries, they are only recognized in that specific state or locality.

Although domestic partnerships and civil unions expand the relatively non-existent rights of same sex couples, they are severely limited alternatives. Supporters of equal rights for gay and lesbian persons contend that the only true way to solidify same sex relationships is via marriage. They argue that any other alternative serves to create second-class relationships, therein fostering the oppression that currently exists.

DISCUSSION

The judicial system has become a fundamental agent in the struggle to secure equal civil rights for gay men, lesbian women, and their families. Social service providers at all levels must be able to dissect judicial decisions into consequential and valuable information. The model presented within this paper can be used by social service practitioners working with gay and lesbian headed families at all levels; including social service educators, social work micro practitioners working with gay men, lesbian women, and their families, as well as those practitioners working on macro levels such as activists and advocates.

The visibility of gay and lesbian headed families is increasing, and it is essential that social service providers be able to provide quality services to gay and lesbian clients and their families. One mandate of social work's mission is to address oppressive structures and processes. One method that may be useful to social service practitioners is to identify the impact of legislative policy on oppressed populations. Social service providers can use the proposed model as a means of dissecting judicial decisions that affect their gay and lesbian clients. In order to alleviate oppression, we must be able to understand how oppressive structures work and the model presented here is designed in a manner that is user-friendly enough that those who are not especially familiar with politics and the judicial process can easily navigate through a case to uncover the values associated and the true policy issues.

Clearly there is much work to be done to combat legislative discrimination and oppression of gay men, lesbians, and their families. Social workers and other social services providers must continue to support legislative initiatives that enhance civil liberties for all citizens, while working to stop those that exclude, or limit the rights of gay men and lesbians. Understanding the facts and implications of judicial decisions such as the *Goodridge* (2003) case is vital.

It is generally believed among social science researchers that rights should be applied equally to all members of society. However, few policy analysis models are designed to fit the unique specifications of thought analysis of court decision. The model presented within this paper carries the analysis through a logical progression of steps designed to establish the factors of the case, identify the policy issue(s), evaluate the supporting and opposing arguments, deconstruct the values at the center of the issue, conduct an interest analysis to determine those affected by the ruling, and consider alternative solutions.

REFERENCES

Cahill, S., & Slater,S. (2004). Legal protections for families and children. *National Gay and Lesbian Task Force Policy Institute: Author.*

Falk, P. (1989). Lesbian mothers psychosocial assumptions in family law. *American Psychologist, 44,* 941-947.

Flaks, D., Ficher, I., Masterpasqua, F., & Joseph, G. (1995). Lesbians choosing motherhood: A comparative study of lesbians and heterosexual parents and their children. *Developmental Psychology, 31*(1), 105-114.

Moroney, R. M. (1981). Policy analysis within a value theoretical framework. In Gallagher, J. J. & Haskins, R. (Eds.). *Models for analysis of social policy: An introduction* (pp. 78-102). Norwood, New Jersey: Ablex Publishing.

Gay and Lesbian Advocates and Defenders. (2007). *Legal issues for non-Massachusetts same-sex couples who married in Massachusetts.* Retrieved April 25, 2007 from the World Wide Web: http://www.glad.org/marriage/outofstate_legalissues. html

Golombock, S., Spencer, A., & Rutter, M. (1983). Children in lesbian and single parent households: Psychosexual and psychiatric appraisal. *Journal of Child Psychology and Psychiatry,* 24, 551-572.

Goodridge v. Department of Public Health, 440 Mass. 309, 798 N.E.2d 941 (2003).

Gottman, J. S. (1990). Children of gay and lesbian parents. In F. W. Bozett & M. B. Sussman, (Eds.), *Homosexuality and family relations* (pp. 177-196). New York: Harrington Park Press.

Green, R., Mandel, J.B., Hotvedt, M. E., Gray, J., & Smith, L. (1986). Lesbian mothers and their children: A comparison with solo parent heterosexual mothers and their children. *Archives of Sexual Behaviors, 15,* 167-184.

Harris, M., & Turner, P. (1985). Gay and lesbian parenting. *Journal of Homosexuality, 12,* 101-113.

Huggins, S. L. (1989). A comparative study of self-esteem of adolescent children of divorced lesbian mothers and divorced heterosexual mothers. In F. W. Bozett (Ed.), *Homosexuality and the family* (pp. 123-135). New York: Harrington Park Press.

Kirkpatrick, M., Smith, C., & Roy, R. (1981). Lesbian mothers and their children: A comparative study. *American Journal of Orthopsychiatry,* 51, 545-551.

Loving v. Virginia, 388 U.S. 1, 87 S. Ct. 1817, 18 L.Ed.2d 1010, U.S. Va. (1967).

Sailer, S. (2003, July). Gay marriage around the globe. *United Press International.* Retrieved April 1, 2004 from *http://www.upi.com/view.cfm/storyID=20030714-073510-5671r.*

Tunbull, H. R. (1981). Two legal analysis techniques and public policy analysis. In Gallagher, J. J. & Haskins, R. (Eds.). *Models for analysis of social policy: An introduction* (pp. 153-173). Norwood, New Jersey: Ablex Publishing.

U.S. Census Bureau. (2000). *Marital status by sex, unmarried-partner households, and grandparents as caregivers: 2000.* Retrieved April 25, 2007 from http://factfinder. census.gov/servlet/QTTable?_bm=y&-geo_id=01000US&-qr_name=DEC_2000_ SF3_U_QTP18&-ds_name=DEC_2000_SF3_U

Zablocki v. Redhail, 434 U.S. 374, 98 S. Ct. 673, 54 L.Ed.2d 618 (1978).

Lesbian Parent Activism and Meaning-Making in the Current Political Environment: One Community's Story

Barbara L. Jones
Tanya M. Voss

At this moment in our political and social history, the rights of lesbian, gay, bisexual and transgender (LGBT) families are being discussed, legislated, and contested like never before. There has been a dramatic increase in political attempts to ban legal recognition of same-sex relationships. By the end of 2006, 27 states had enacted constitutional amendments banning same-sex marriage and 41 states had legislated that marriage can only exist between a man and woman. At the same time, a few states seem to be moving towards acknowledging same-sex relationships. The state of Massachusetts became the first in the nation to issue marriage licenses to same-sex couples in 2004. As recently as February 2007, New Jersey became the third state to approve civil unions, behind Vermont in 2000 and Connecticut in 2005 . This was the result of a New Jersey Supreme Court ruling in *Lewis v. Harris* that same-sex couples have a constitutional right to the same state benefits, protections and responsibilities as opposite-sex married couples (New York Times, February 20, 2007). However, most of the political activity has served to limit benefits and rights for LGBT families. In many communities in the United States, LGBT community members and their allies have organized community responses to the political and social attacks on their families. Since much of the legislation affects family life, there has been a preponderance of LGBT-headed households involved in these activist efforts. This community activism has resulted in political successes and setbacks (Bonelli, 2004; Grise-Owens, 2004; McClellan & Greif, 2004; Otis, 2004; Padilla, 2004). Regardless of the outcome of the activism, the actions themselves may have an effect the participants. While recognizing the efforts of the entire LGBT community in these actions, this article will focus on the lesbian parents who have become involved in activism. Both the potential motivations for this activism and the potential effects on lesbian parents will be discussed in this article, using the case of Austin, Texas, as one example.

LESBIAN PARENTED FAMILIES

The 2000 U.S. Census report on Married-Couple and Unmarried-Partner Households estimates the number of same-sex partner households at 594,391 nationwide. Of these households, 293,365 or 49.4% percent were female couples. In fact, the 1990 census was the first time the Census Bureau listed "unmarried partner" as an option on the census form. According to those data, 150,000 people reported being in same-sex couples in households located in 52% of all U.S. counties. Due at least in part to more accurate systems in 2000, the census reports that same-sex couples reside in 99.3% of all US counties. The census reports that 34% of female same-sex headed households and 22% of male ones included children (U.S. Census, 2000). The number of children living in LGBT-headed households is difficult to estimate but various reports estimate that 6 to 12 million children are living with at least one gay or lesbian parent (Human Rights Campaign, 2006; Patterson, 1992).

Lesbian-headed families are a remarkably heterogeneous group and can include single parents, partnered parents and married parents. The children being raised by lesbian parents include biological children from previous relationships, children who are born in prior or current same-sex coupled relationships, and children who are fostered and/or adopted into the family. This wide range of family constellations, coupled with the homophobia which causes many lesbian parents to hide their true relationship, makes accurate estimates and descriptions of lesbian-headed families difficult to obtain.

Similar problems exist in studying the children of lesbian-headed families (Meezan & Rauch, 2005). However, most of the research that has been done on same-sex parents has been conducted on lesbian-headed households (Meezan & Rauch, 2005). The evidence from these studies shows that children raised by lesbian mothers are not statistically different from other children. The American Psychological Association (2004) states "that the development, adjustment, and well-being of children with lesbian and gay parents does not differ markedly from that of children with heterosexual parents" (www.apa.org). Lesbian and gay-headed families are also supported by the American Psychiatric Association, American Academy of Pediatrics, American Sociological Association, Child Welfare League of America, and the American Academy of Family Physicians, the American Academy of Child & Adolescent Psychiatry, and the National Association of Social Workers. Despite this widespread professional and empirical support, lesbian-headed households face societal and legislative challenges to their families every day.

Scope of the Impact and Threats

In 2003, the U.S. Supreme Court ruled *Lawrence v. Texas* unconstitutional and broadened the realm of action and discussion about what the ruling called the declaration of the dignity of homosexual citizens. Robertson states,

> Past struggles for gay and lesbian rights have confronted criminal bans on gay sexuality and discrimination in employment, the military, and other areas of public life. With *Lawrence v. Texas* having struck down laws against sodomy, the front lines of the struggle for gay rights have moved to issues of same-sex marriage and child-rearing. (Robertson, 2004, p. 324)

A few months later in the same year, the Massachusetts Supreme Judicial Court upheld the right to same-sex marriage in the landmark *Goodridge v. Department of Public Health* ruling. This paved the way for the country's first same-sex marriages in 2004. The national and state-by-state debate about marriage and relationship recognition for lesbian and gay-headed households has been intense ever since. As Robertson notes,

> The issue of same-sex marriage has reminded the country that gays and lesbians often have and rear offspring. Indeed, gay and lesbian parenting of children was a driving force in Massachusetts' landmark legal recognition of same-sex marriage. As more gays and lesbians enter into partnership arrangements, a growing number will seek to have children. (Robertson, 2004, p. 324)

Prior to 2004, only a handful of states had constitutional language defining marriage as exclusively between a man and a woman. A flurry of legislative activity, however, has translated into 27 states with constitutional bans on same-sex marriage as of November 2006, with some states' language going further to prevent anything "identical or similar to marriage." Arizona is the only state to defeat a proposed constitutional ban on same-sex marriage. Forty-one states have legislative statutes defining marriage as between one woman and one man (Human Rights Campaign, 2006). As of this writing, ten state legislatures have marriage amendment initiatives pending in their legislatures (Human Rights Campaign, 2006). Additionally, the U.S. also has the military's "Don't Ask, Don't Tell, Don't Pursue" which applies to the homosexual conduct and relationships of its service members (1993) and a federal Defense of Marriage Act (1996).

Marriage as a legal institution affords 1,138 different legal protections and responsibilities to its participants (U.S. General Accounting Office, 2004). These include divorce, social security benefits, health care benefits and decision-making power, inheritance laws and the right to decline to testify in court against a spouse, to name a few. Many of these legal designations and guidelines are about property. These rights and responsibilities disproportionately affect lesbian parents because of the difference in earnings women typically face. Women working full-time earn an average of 80 cents for every dollar men earn (U.S. General Accounting Office, 2004). For example, when a married parent dies, the remaining parent receives benefits through the social security office to offset the cost of raising a child. An unmarried partner, even in second-parent adoptions, does not receive that benefit, which can amount to many hundreds of dollars a month. This benefit is a property resource that, if available, is designed to acknowledge and supplement the child's need in light of the loss of the deceased parent. It is a resource not available to same-sex couples because they cannot wed or, if they do, the federal Defense of Marriage Act (1996) prevents federal recognition and benefits associated with their marriage.

Foster Care and Adoption

Rulings and legislation regarding lesbians and gays as parents have implications for existing same-sex headed households related to second-parent adoptions by same-sex persons, custody issues, school relationships and hospital visitation policies. Lesbian parents have not historically received the benefits of legislation and policy on any of these issues but neither have they been the focus of so much activity around defining and restricting rights and relationships.

Additionally, the rights of lesbians and gay men to adopt or foster children have been significantly challenged in many states at a time when the need for adoptive and foster families in this country is in critical shortage. The U.S. Department of Health and Human Services Administration for Children and Families Adoption and Foster Care Analysis and Reporting System 2000 estimates state that there are approximately 520,000 children in foster care in the United States. Of these, 117,000 are eligible for adoption and about half of these are racial and ethnic minorities (US HHS, 2000).

While currently eight states and the District of Columbia allow second-parent adoptions officially and fifteen states allow second-parent adoption in some jurisdictions, four states have court rulings that disallow second-parent adoptions (Human Rights Campaign, 2006). Florida officially prohibits single LGBT persons from adopting or fostering children and North Dakota, Nebraska, Missouri, and Arkansas statutes are unclear as to whether they will allow single LGBT persons to adopt (Human Rights Campaign, 2006). A number of states, including Texas, Georgia and Kansas, have recently proposed initiatives to prohibit single LGBT persons from adopting or fostering children.

In Texas, legislation has been introduced every session since 1999 that would deny otherwise qualified and agency-approved lesbian or gay people from becoming foster or adoptive parents. In this same state, there were 27,931 children in the foster care system in 2004 with only 680 foster homes available (Department of Family and Protective Services, 2004). Texas is one of seven states to introduce bills like this in 2005. Ohio is moving forward in seeking a ban on gays and lesbians from being foster or adoptive parents in 2006 (Christian Science Monitor, 2006). These legislative efforts occur despite rulings like *Goodridge v. Department of Public Health* in Massachusetts that stated that the state's ban on same-sex marriage was not rationally related to its legitimate goal of protecting the interest of children. Efforts to restrict same-sex couples legalizing of their family structure have the potential to actually harm family stability and children's' legal protection. As Robertson (2004) writes,

> Excluding same-sex couples from civil marriage will not make children of opposite sex marriages more secure, but it does prevent children of same-sex couples from enjoying the immeasurable advantages that flow from the assurance of "a stable family structure in which children will be reared, educated, and socialized. (p. 324)

Activism as a Form of Meaning-Making

Given the demands of parenthood and the current hostile political climate, it is curious that lesbian parents engage in activism at all. Understanding this activity and identifying potential positive benefits can help community organizers, clinicians, and lesbian parents and their children. Activism may provide a context for lesbian parents to develop community, create meaning, enhance self-esteem, identify allies, and, when successful, prepare for and protect their children from harmful legislation.

One framework for understanding lesbian parent activism is to look at it as a response to the trauma of societal and political homophobia. Trauma occurs when an individual is exposed to a stressful event that they cannot escape and that is overwhelming to their coping mechanisms (Van der Kolk et al, 1996). A steady stream of homophobic messages, actions, and policies certainly constitutes exposure to stress that is inescapable for lesbian-headed households. Homophobia has the potential to cause psychological and sometimes physical injury to lesbian parents and their children (Perrin & Kulkin, 1996; Speziale & Gopalakrishna, 2004; Stein, Perrin & Potter, 2004).

Traumatized individuals may choose to react by withdrawing, hiding or retreating (flight) or by standing up to (fight) the forces that are trying to oppress them. Choosing to fight involves a deliberate plan to face fear and perhaps danger and then to take intentional action (Herman, 1992). For lesbian parents, taking a stance publicly is definitely a conscious choice that requires understanding the potential risk of harm to their family. Choosing to act may itself have a positive impact on surviving the trauma of homophobic and heterosexist societal and legislative acts. Both the grief and trauma literature have identified "taking action" as a tool for healing from and transcending trauma and loss (Herman, 1992; McCann & Perlman, 1990; Neimeyer, 2001). According to McCann and Perlman (1990), factors that predict trauma survival include: having a meaningful community where one can self-disclose, having a sense of identity, and engaging in pro-social behavior including efforts to create societal change. Community activism can immediately provide those involved with a sense of community and identity. By engaging in community activism, lesbian parents may experience a solidarity and sense of belonging and validation at a time when they are being politically and socially disenfranchised. Some research has already described how lesbian parents' involvement in their children's schools is beneficial to the family and the community (Mercier & Harold, 2003). Perhaps the activism provides an antidote for lesbian parents to the isolation and trauma of cultural messages and social policies that seek to invalidate and in some cases cause direct harm to their families.

Another perspective which may explain the involvement of lesbian parents in community activism is a social constructionist theory of responding to loss. Social constructivism states that meaning in life is cognitively created or constructed by individuals in a social context. In fact, many social work and psychology theorists have begun to discuss meaning making or meaning reconstruction as a part of psychological growth and resilience (Armour, 2002; Greene, 2002; Neimeyer, 2001), Parenting in a hostile environment can create both primary and secondary losses for lesbian parents and their children. Primary losses can include: loss of jobs, loss of school, loss of community, loss of custody, loss of family support, loss of health benefits, and loss of financial security. Secondary losses can include: loss of self esteem, loss of sense of safety, loss of sense of control, loss of hope, loss of freedom, or loss of belief in a just world, and loss of spiritual faith and support. These losses are an additional burden on lesbian parent families as compared to their heterosexual counterparts.

All families construct meanings of their experiences and their place in the world. For families facing loss, threat or challenge, meanings have to be reconstructed in order for the family to survive the loss (Nadeau, 2001). For lesbian-headed families, getting involved in community activism may serve the function of meaning reconstruction so that they can envision their families contextually as supported, loved and capable of responding to threat.

Other family groups that have faced threat or loss have utilized action as a form of coping with their distress. In a study of homicide survivor families, Armour (2003) found that surviving trauma sometimes means moving past a cognitive reconstruction to a performative dimension of meaning-making. One of the findings of this study was that homicide survivor families described a meaning making grounded in action (Armour, 2003) where pursuing what mattered provided a form of coping that involved taking conscious and intentional actions that had personal and symbolic meaning. For lesbian families, an "intense pursuit of what matters" may serve a number of psychological functions. First, it may provide a sense of a survivor self-identity as the parents take deliberate action to counteract attempts to limit their families' rights. Secondly, the pursuit itself could create an opportunity for lesbian-headed households to speak the truth of their families in the face of many politically motivated misconceptions and misstatements. And third, having a pursuit may offer a prosocial activity in which to channel sadness, anger, hurt, and loss while creating positive social change.

ONE COMMUNITY'S STORY

In Austin, Texas, two lesbian mothers formed a grassroots coalition, The Austin Alliance for Social Justice, in response to efforts to ban same-sex marriage in their state. This coalition not only contributed to the defeat of the ban in one Texas County but also led to other efforts that positively impacted LGBT civil rights in Central Texas. One of the founders of the Austin Alliance for Social Justice stated, "We just felt that somebody had to do something–*we* had to do something. We could not just let them continue to pass legislation against our families without standing up and fighting, without saying, without screaming that it is wrong to do this to people and to families. I'd rather go down swinging that sit here passively and let them insult us and our children. We are doing what any good parent would do–fighting to protect our children who are under attack" (S. Marriott, personal communication, June 14, 2005).

In May, 2005, the Texas Legislature passed for public vote what would become Proposition 2. When it reached the ballot in November, the proposition read

> The constitutional amendment providing that marriage in this state consists only of the union of one man and one woman and prohibiting this state or a political subdivision of this state from creating or recognizing any legal status identical or similar to marriage. (Texas Legislative Council, 2007)

On June 5, Governor Rick Perry signed the bill at the Calvary Christian Academy gymnasium even though his signature was not necessary in moving the language forward to Texas voters. At that press conference, a reporter asked the governor what he would tell gay and lesbian veterans currently fighting the war on terror overseas when they returned if this amendment passed. The governor replied as if the outcome of the impending vote was a foregone conclusion, "Texans have made a decision about marriage and if there is some other state that has a more lenient view than Texas then maybe that's a better place for them to live" (The Washington Post, p. A18, June 18, 2005)

In the capitol city of Austin, two lesbian moms decided that it was time to take action. It was one thing to be disregarded by Texas' law. It was another to have their scant legal protections undermined by the governor and a constitutional amendment that not only excluded them from marriage but also called into question the limited legal parameters they had been able to piece together. On June 18, the couple hosted 28 community leaders in their living room. The guests were invited for their proven leadership, commitment and/or energy for a diverse LGBT community. A flip chart welcomed people with Margaret Meade's statement: "Never doubt that a small committed group of citizens can change the world. In fact, it is the only thing that ever has." The hosts, a couple of almost 17 years and mothers of two young boys, provided brunch and coffee, a challenge to hope, a call to action and a commitment to listening. The sign-in sheet and handout headings read "Operation Hope."

The couple opened the meeting with an acknowledgement of the hurt, despair and anger they had been hearing. Some in the community were talking about flight to other states. The majority of people were shrugging a helpless resignation to the amendment's passage; it was Texas after all. A few were ready to fight and take action but did not know where to start. This couple decided to fight and asked who would join in. At the very least, they could work to hold Austin Travis County as a beacon of hope for lesbians and gays across the state. This vision came out of the group's meeting:

> We're clear that we're committed to peacefully and passionately fighting the oppressive constitutional amendment that's in front of us. We're clear that we will win the fight to gain ground and community over the next 20 weeks. We're clear that this loose coalition is one voice representing an important part of the energy and diversity of our community that remains committed to the overall unified goal of securing our rights. (Austin Alliance for Social Justice, June 18, 2006)

The leaders collected 58 written pledges for specific action that day. Commitments included everything from agreeing to one-on-one conversations with people who might not know how this legislation would hurt the speaker personally, to donating free copy services, attending the next meeting, developing voter pledge cards, hosting house parties, and organizing a vigil.

Remarkably, just thirteen days later, this group did host a community vigil at the State capitol. The flier read, "This year, start your 4th of July weekend by joining gay and straight fair-minded Texans for a vigil at the Capitol. Veterans will lead the way as we walk together to the Capitol to protest Governor Perry's outrageous insult to Texas' brave and heroic LGBT service members. We are also praying for added strength and hope for the thousands of LGBT individuals and families that would be harmed by passage of the shameful anti-gay constitutional amendment on the ballot in Texas this November."

A retired Army chaplain colonel provided the emotional lead in organizing the vigil and enlisted the aid of two LGBT veteran groups to provide the color guard and 200 individual U.S. flags. The host couple covered the costs and logistics associated with permits and equipment. Another lesbian mom couple secured the support of a sponsoring legislator's office. One of the gay dads helped the group envision and enact not a rally but a vigil based on the non-violent principles and teachings of Gandhi and Martin Luther King, Jr. promoted by the organization Soulforce. Many other volunteers were involved in media contacts, flier distribution and crowd direction.

The local newspaper, *The Austin-American Statesman,* reported 300 people standing in silent vigil encircling the capitol building and the action was covered by every local news station (The Austin-American Statesman, July 2, 2005). The name of the organization grew up as organically as the group itself had. Members of the vigil committee were required to fill in the sponsoring organization blank on the permits and came up with The Austin Alliance for Social Justice. The name stuck.

The next meeting brought in 46 people including the creative director for a major advertising firm in town. The creative director and her two small children had been at the original couple's house for hamburgers and hot dogs one night when the conversation turned to the proposed amendment and the meeting this couple had hosted. Their children all played together regularly at each others' houses and went to school together. She knew her neighbors as a lesbian-headed family but said that not until that night and seeing the tears in her friends' eyes did she "get it." She said she wanted in on the fight to help other married people like her understand the personal cost to real people, too. She became an active part of the Alliance and spearheaded the development and donation of a $150,000 educational digital video disc that was used statewide for educational and fundraising purposes. The "No Nonsense in November" statewide campaign name was born from the brainstorming that the creative director facilitated at the second meeting.

The newly formed steering committee recognized that the group had outgrown the living room and found a church to host the third Alliance meeting. This church had never before hosted or sponsored an LGBT-focused event but on a Saturday in July, it opened its doors to 62 people engaged in the Alliance. The fourth meeting was held at a different church, this time recruited by another lesbian mom couple. At this meeting, the Alliance founders introduced more than 100 attendees to the statewide "No Nonsense in November" Travis County coordinating team, some of whom had been active with the Alliance from the beginning. As a result of this meeting, activists distributed voter pledge cards, deputized approximately 50 voter registrars, sold the newly designed t-shirts and collected $4,800 for the statewide campaign.

The Alliance remained active throughout the campaign in mobilizing volunteers, coordinating with allied organizations, voter identification and registration, and get-out-the-vote activities. Alliance members organized three vigils and one multi-faith service, produced and distributed the DVD statewide for educational and fundraising purposes, kept an up to date website and developed and distributed church bulletin inserts to churches and neighborhoods. The second vigil's focus was "Love Your Neighbors–All of Them" and representatives from the Alliance and the Travis County "No Nonsense in November" office spoke at neighborhood association meetings about Proposition 2 in preparation for the vigil and the vote. Over the course of the campaign, ten Austin-based faith communities were newly identified and mobilized as supporting equal rights for LGBT persons and their families.

All these activities were in coordination and cooperation with many other organizations and citizens from across the state and Travis County including Atticus Circle, The University of Texas' Campus Alliance Against Inequality, the Lesbian Gay Rights Lobby, Texas Freedom Network, PFLAG (Parents and Friends of Lesbians and Gays), and many other like-minded groups. Many organizations did not join in. Activists were frustrated by the limited support from national LGBT rights groups and the lackluster involvement of non-gay groups including Democratic clubs. The local organization for LGBT people of color, ALLGO, was in transition with its leadership during the campaign and that transition impacted their level of participation.

The LGBT parenting community in Austin has in its brief history been minimally organized but exclusively around social events such as play dates. As a group, none of these informal organizations picked up the challenge of political activism. As individuals and families, many were involved in many ways including rallies, block walking and providing babysitting to those parents who were involved. The formation of the Austin Alliance for Social Justice marked the first time in this community that lesbian, gay, bisexual and transgender parents were central to an organized political fight against legislation aimed at their families.

As is often the case, political activism does not come without cost. In the fall of 2005, two events occurred that highlighted the danger and fear that many LGBT activists were facing. In September, a member of the Alliance steering committee and chair of the statewide faith committee was assaulted in his home. Police classified the attack as a hate crime after the election based on the homophobic slurs prevalent during the assault. Four lesbian mom couples pitched in and sent flowers on behalf of the Alliance. Then, three days before the November 8 election, the Ku Klux Klan held its first Austin-based rally in 35 years for the explicit purpose of supporting family values by encouraging voters to vote yes on the anti-gay amendment. The Alliance chose not to participate as a group in the counter protest because it did not want to give any energy or attention to the KKK. However, the presence of the group in Austin brought home the chilling reality of the inherent dangers whenever a socially disenfranchised group organizes for rights.

On November 8th, the day of the election, Alliance members spent hours distributing door hangers, standing on street corners with home-made posters, phone banking, talking to family and friends, and voting. In other Texas counties, volunteers at the polls were dodging signs ripped out of the ground and thrown at them, as well as homophobic epithets. In Austin, a crowd of activists and stakeholders gathered at a local restaurant to watch the results come in election night. The results were clear as soon as the polls closed–perhaps the only real suspense had ever been the margin. The amendment passed 76-24 percent statewide. In some counties, it passed 95-5 percent. By a 60-40 split, Travis County was the one county of all Texas' 254 that defeated Prop 2. Despite the statewide defeat, this was a significant win for Travis County and for Texas. Still, no one was celebrating the night of November 8, 2005. Activists who had fought so hard to defeat Proposition 2 were saddened by its passage. However, after a period of quiet, the Austin Alliance for Social Justice reorganized and is now involved in other efforts to promote civil rights for LGBT families in Central Texas.

Proposition 2 was the critical incident that helped the Austin LGBT community organize. The Alliance continues beyond the election with a new and expanded steering committee. Their mission:

> To support and preserve American social justice as it specifically relates to equal rights for people of all sexual orientations within the Central Texas/Austin area.

The Alliance has adopted a focus on building an LGBT community ready for action in support of LGBT rights with an extra emphasis on bridging to non-traditional allies such as communities of color, heterosexual communities, veterans and communities of faith. The instigating lesbian parent couple remain involved but the new facilitator for meetings and discussions is another lesbian mom, one who is motivated to activism by the loss of her children to her ex-husband because of her sexual orientation.

The Alliance continued to be involved in community activist events related to rights for LGBT persons and their families. The Alliance contributed to coalition efforts in May 2006 that resulted in the City of Austin removing a prohibition related to health insurance. The citizens of Austin voted that "The City Charter be amended to restore a city employee's ability to purchase additional benefit coverage." The Austin City Council has not yet instated this benefit coverage at the date of this writing, but it now has the freedom to offer benefits to a city employee's designated household member including, but not limited to, a same-sex partner.

FUTURE IMPLICATIONS

Many communities in the United States have been organizing to fight discrimination against lesbian, gay, bisexual and transgender families. This story was not unique in that way. What was notable about the Austin effort is that it began in the living room of two Texan lesbian moms, two community members who had not previously been motivated to organize this way, and that it was sustained in large part by others like them fighting for marriage and family. It came out of their anger at being misrepresented, their desire to act and their need to protect their children. Out of this simple effort at community organizing, a new organization was formed to continue to fight for social justice in Austin, a discriminatory measure was plainly defeated in Austin's home county, a community was inspired and individuals were uplifted even in defeat.

In this community, lesbian parents led the struggle to fight political institutions that would limit their families' rights to healthcare, financial security, and legal protections. The interaction between lesbian parents and the political environment has been little studied. Implications for research include qualitative studies of lesbian parent activists and their children regarding the meaning of being involved politically and quantitative studies to assess the number and impact of lesbian mother political activists. Researchers may need to catalog and describe the activism of lesbian and gay parents as the struggle for social justice continues. The history of the movement for marriage, adoption, and family equality can and should be documented by social scientists. Additionally, social science researchers have a responsibility to raise legitimate scientific concern about questionable research that inaccurately represents the attributes and outcomes of same-sex headed families. The current court of public opinion often clamors for two sides to every politically sensitive story and this can create an environment in which less rigorous research is allowed to circulate.

Lesbian parents offer a unique voice to the struggle for equality and social justice for LGBT families. By organizing their communities, they may create positive social change and impact their own emotional well-being and that of their families. Social service practitioners at all levels should explore the involvement of lesbian parents in activism to include this as a part of the web of meaning for these families. Clinicians working with lesbian parents may find that their clients need and want to discuss their desires and fears about involving themselves in political activities. For those lesbian parents who do engage in activism, it is important for practitioners to inquire about this aspect of their identity and help to integrate that into other aspects of identity such as mother, partner, daughter, employee, friend. For those lesbian parents who identify political activism as too risky or dangerous for them based on their community, their work, or their children's needs, clinicians can respect and support these decisions. Clinicians should do so from an informed stance based on current research regarding parent activism and current information about activities happening in their communities. Stories of other parents organizing can create solidarity and hope for those who may not have the ability to join in that type of effort or perhaps for those who have never considered such activities for themselves. Identifying and understanding the activism that lesbian parents engage in may provide a place to discuss issues of isolation and community, defeat and hope, tragedy and personal growth. The empowerment benefit of community organizing and activism is an understudied aspect of lesbian parent life that clinicians and researchers should address in the future.

Lesbian parents who engage in activism in their communities must fully assess the risk to themselves and their children and practitioners can help them do this. For those in Austin, there was legitimate parental concern about how being on the front lines of such visible activism would affect the children, and parents made efforts to prepare and protect the children. Parents talked with each other about ways to let children be a part of what was happening in an age-appropriate way. For example, a six-year-old boy whose lesbian parents were active was heard telling his friends that the campaign was a "fight between the mom-and-dad families and families like ours." His parents responded by talking with him but also by intentionally inviting friends who were "mom-and-dad families" with children their son's age to show up at different events in support of "families like ours."

Some parents chose to keep their children out of public events altogether. Most parents found ways to shield their children from the negative commentary of the opposition that was often evident in media reports, i.e., not watching the news with video and commentary on the children and their families. Some parents used the community organizing to open up discussions of rights and freedom and family. Some allied heterosexual parents also used the community events as an opportunity to show solidarity and to teach their own children about social justice. Parents also were referred to online resources on how to talk to children about the current political climate (Family Pride Coalition, 2006). Parents who have any reason to fear oppression learn ways to protect their children. The LGBT parents in Austin made very personal choices about this based on experience, comfort, legal status of parental rights, developmental stages and individual needs of the children and personal feelings of safety. Clinicians and community organizers must recognize that lesbian parents who engage in activism need support, education and preparation about how to protect their children.

Community organizers might also begin to approach the fight for social justice as one that has implicit benefits to the community regardless of outcome. Even when community organizing efforts do not reach their ultimate goal, as in Texas, smaller goals may be reached. This concept, sometimes referred to as "losing forward" refers to the ability of a social movement to use defeats as an opportunity to move the entire community forward toward the ultimate goal of social justice (Wolfson, 2004). In Austin, Travis County defeated Proposition 2 in opposition to the rest of the state. This created energy amongst the activists for continued efforts towards social change. The Austin Alliance for Social Justice has continued to function as a presence in the Austin community with a current database of approximately 300 people active during and since the amendment fight.

The political and societal attention on lesbian, gay, bisexual and transgender families is continuing as is evidenced by the pending legislative restrictions regarding foster care and adoption. This makes understanding the social, political and personal impact of activism critical to lesbian parents in their social environment. Lesbian parent activism may contribute to defeating anti-gay political legislation in various communities around the United States. Perhaps more importantly, the actions themselves may help lesbian parents and their children form alliances, feel supported, build community, enhance self-esteem, empower themselves and begin to heal from societal homophobia.

REFERENCES

American Psychological Association (2004). Resolution on sexual orientation, parents and children. Retrieved April 4, 2006 from http://www.apa.org/pi/reslgbc.html

Armour, M. (2002). Meaning making in the aftermath of homicide. *Death Studies., 27,* 519-540.

Austin Alliance for Social Justice (2006) personal communication, June 18, 2006

Austin-American Statesman (July 2, 2005). Gay, lesbians hold march, 'equality vigil' at Capitol.

Bennett, L. & Gates, G.J. (2004). The cost of marriage inequality to children and their same-sex parents. A Human Rights Campaign Foundation report. Retrieved April 4, 2006 from www.hrc.org.

Bonelli, J. & Simmons, L. (2004). Coalition building and electoral organizing in the passage of anti-discrimination laws: The case of Connecticut. *Journal of Gay and Lesbian Social Services, 16*(3.4), 35-53.

Family Pride Coalition–Raising your Family (2006) Retrieved April 1, 2006 from http://www.familypride.org/site/pp.asp?c=bhKPI7PFImE&b=392245

Greene, R. R. (Ed.). (2002). *Resilience: An integrated approach to practice, policy and research.* Washington, D.C.: N.A.S.W. Press.

Grise-Owens, E., Vessels, J. & Owens, L.W. (2004). Building coalitions and changing communities organizing for change: One city's journey toward justice. *Journal of Gay and Lesbian Social Services, 16*(3/4), 1-15.

Herman, J. L. (1992). *Trauma and recovery: The aftermath of violence from domestic abuse to political terror.* New York, New York: Basic Books.

Human Rights Campaign–Laws and Legislation in Your State (2006) Retrieved November 8, 2006fromhttp://www.hrc.org/Template.cfm?Section=Your_Community&Template=/ContentManagement/ContentDisplay.cfm&ContentID=8471

Marriott, S., personal communication, June 14, 2005.

McCann, I. L. & Pearlman, L.A. (1990). *Psychological, trauma and the adult survivor: Theory, therapy and transformation.* New York, New York: Brunner/Mazel, Inc.

McClellan, D. L. & Greif, G.L. (2004). Organizing to amend antidiscrimination statutes in Maryland. *Journal of Gay and Lesbian Social Services, 16*(3/4), 55-68.

Meezan, W. & Rauch, J. (2005). Gay marriage, same-sex parenting, and America's children. *Future Child., 15*(2), 97-115.

Mercier, L. R. a. H., R.D. (2003). At the interface: Lesbian-parent families and their children's schools. *Children and Schools, 25*(1), 35-37.

Nadeau, J. W. (2001). Family construction of meaning. In R. A. E. Neimeyer (Ed.), *Meaning reconstruction and the experience of loss* (Vol. 95-111). Washington, D.C.: N.A.S.W. Press.

Neimeyer, R. A. (Ed.). (2001). *Meaning reconstruction and the experience of loss.* Washington, D.C.: American Psychological Association.

New York Times (February 20, 2007). Eagerness and some resignation as civil union law takes effect.

Otis, M. (2004). One community's path to greater social justice: Building on earlier successes. *Journal of Gay and Lesbian Social Services, 16*(3/4), 17-33.

Padilla, Y. C. (Ed.). (2004). *Gay and lesbian rights organizing: Community based strategies.* Binghamton, New York: Harrington Park Press.

Patterson, C. (1992). Children of lesbian and gay parents. *Child Development,* (63), 1025-1042.

Perrin, E.C. and Kulkin, H. (1996). Pediatric care for children whose parents are gay or lesbian. *Pediatrics,* 97, 629-635

Robertson, J.A. (2004). Gay and lesbian access to assisted reproductive technology. *Case Western Reserve Law Review.* 55(2), 323-372.

Speziale, B. and Gopalakrishna, V. (2004). Social support and functioning of nuclear families headed by lesbian couples. *Affilia,* 19 (2), 178-184.

Stein, M.T., Perrin, E.C, and Potter, J. (2004). A difficult adjustment to school: The importance of family constellation. *Pediatrics,* 114 (5), 1464-1467.

Texas Legislative Council. (2007). *Analyses of proposed constitutional amendments (p.17).* Retrieved online March 6, 2007 fromhttp://www.sos.state.tx.us/elections/voter/2005novconsamend.shtml.

U.S. General Accounting Office (2004) Defense of Marriage Act, GAO/OGC-97-16, January 31, 1997 and GAO-04-353R updated January 23, 2004.

U.S. Department of Health and Human Services, Administration for Children and Families, Administration on Children, Youth and Families, Children's Bureau. (2000, January). *Current estimates as of January 2000* (Rep. No. 2). Washington, D.C.: U.S. Department of Health and Human Services. Retrieved April 9, 2006, from http://www.acf.hhs.gov/programs/cb/stats_research/afcars/tar/report2/ar0100a.htm

U.S. Census Bureau. (2000). *Marital Status by Sex, Unmarried-Partner Households,* and Grandparents as Caregivers: 2000. Retrieved April 9, 2006 from http://factfinder.census.gov/servlet/QTTable?_bm=y&-geo_id=01000US&-qr_name=DEC_2000_SF3_U_QTP18&-ds_name=DEC_2000_SF3_U&-redoLog=false&-format=&-CONTEXT=qt

Van der Kolk, B. A. & McFarlane, A.C. and Weisaeth (Ed.). (1996). *Traumatic stress: The effects of overwhelming experience on mind, body and society.* New York, New York: The Guilford Press.

The Washington Post (June 18, 2005). Commentary: Dishonoring Texas veterans.

Wolfson, E. (2004). *Marriage equality and some lessons for the scary work of winning.* Paper presented at the Lavender Law September 2004: NLGLA's annual gathering of attorneys, legal academics, and law students.

How Heterosexism Plagues Practitioners in Services for Lesbians and Their Families: An Exploratory Study

Sandra C. Anderson
Mindy Holliday

This article addresses the prevalence of heterosexism and homophobia among mental health practitioners who identify as qualified providers for lesbians and their families. In approaching this topic, it is useful to differentiate between homophobia and heterosexism. Homophobia, coined by Weinberg (1972), is an unsatisfactory term for several reasons. First, it is not a real phobia in the clinical sense and second, it implies that personal rather than political solutions are needed to eradicate negative attitudes. In essence, as noted by Kitzinger (1996), the term depoliticizes oppression "by suggesting that the oppression of lesbians comes from the personal inadequacy of particular individuals suffering from a diagnosable phobia" (p. 36). Herek (1996) views the phenomenon as a social one, "rooted in cultural ideologies and inter group relations" (p. 102). He also sees homophobia resulting from heterosexism.

Heterosexism is defined as a belief system in which heterosexuality is seen as superior to and/or more "natural" than homosexuality (Morin, 1997). It is an ideological system that denigrates any non-heterosexual form of behavior or relationship (Herek, 1996). Both homophobia and heterosexism exist in passive (internal) and active (external) forms, and operate on the individual, institutional, and societal levels (see Gruskin, 1999). As heterosexuality is seen as normative, so are traditional gender roles. Gender refers to socially constructed characteristics that express femininity (associated with females) and masculinity (associated with males). Gender expression refers to how a person outwardly manifests gender. Homophobia reinforces traditional gender roles, and intolerance for gender nonconformity is an integral part of heterosexism. Because of this, those who are nonconforming in behavior or appearance are stigmatized.

Lesbians are affected by heterosexism as well as by internalized homophobia. Negative attitudes of clients and therapists toward their own lesbianism, much of which is unrecognized, is reportedly experienced in varying degrees by almost all lesbians raised in a heterosexist society (Cabaj, 2000). Because the authors believe that the client can go only as far in therapy as the therapist herself has gone, it follows that unexamined internalized homophobia can render the therapist unable to effectively work with this issue in clients' lives. Buloff and Osterman (1995) note that the therapist's unexamined heterosexism is potentially more damaging to the lesbian client than overt prejudice.

Heterosexist bias has been found to be common among mental health providers. Garnets, Hancock, Cochran, Goodchilds, and Peplau's (1991) study of 2544 members of the American Psychological Association revealed that many psychologists viewed lesbianism as a psychological disorder, assumed all clients were heterosexual, discouraged or trivialized lesbian experiences, assumed that lesbians have poor parenting skills, and sometimes taught inaccurate information to students. Fourteen percent of the lesbians in Morgan's study (1997) had not sought counseling because they did not know where or how to find a therapist, but believed they would be better off not receiving counseling if the provider were heterosexist.

The correlates of negative attitudes and behavior toward lesbians and gay men have remained fairly consistent over time. As summarized by Herek (1996), those with negative attitudes are less likely to have had personal contact with lesbians or gay men, more likely to report being strongly religious and to subscribe to a conservative religious ideology. They were also more likely to support traditional gender roles, to be older and less well educated, to be more authoritarian, and more likely to have resided in rural areas of the mid-western or southern United States. In addition, heterosexual males tend to manifest higher levels of prejudice than do heterosexual females, especially toward gay men.

A study of undergraduate and graduate social work students (Black, Oles, & Moore, 1998) found a significant relationship between homophobia and sexism, with male students more homophobic and sexist than female students. This is supportive of other findings that negative attitudes toward lesbians and gay men have been consistently linked to negative attitudes toward women and racial and ethnic minorities, suggesting that the dynamics of prejudice are similar across categories (Kite, 1994). Van Wormer (2004) argues that:

> Of all the forms of oppression, the oppression of gender non-conformity is perhaps the most virulent. Unlike other victims of acts of prejudice and discrimination, sexual minorities are taunted on the basis of behavioral characteristics and inclinations that are

thought to be freely chosen . . . Lesbians suffer a double whammy from homophobia because of its link with sexism. (p. 66-67)

Schatz and O'Hanlan (1994) studied lesbian, gay, and bisexual physicians and medical students, and found that 67% knew of patients who had received substandard care because of their sexual orientation, and 88% had heard their colleagues disparage their sexual minority patients. A 1999 study of second year medical students found that 25% viewed homosexuality as "immoral and dangerous to the institution of the family" (Klamen, Grossman, & Kopacz, 1999). The Healthy People 2010 project (2001) reviews the numerous barriers to health care for LGBT people, including provider bias and discrimination. This document also addresses the lack of training provided to medical professionals on how to overcome biases.

Harris, Nightengale, and Owen (1995) found that psychologists and social workers were more educated about homosexuality and had more positive attitudes about lesbians and gay men than did nurses. A 1997 study of MSW social workers (Berkman & Zinberg) found that 10% of respondents were homophobic and the majority was heterosexist. Women were significantly less heterosexist than men, and religiosity was associated with higher levels of homophobia and heterosexism. Knowing a gay man or lesbian and having been in psychotherapy were associated with more positive attitudes.

Saulnier and Wheeler (2000), as part of a larger study, examined lesbians' mental health care in Western New York, and their findings did not support earlier ones. A great majority of respondents (83%) said they were out to their providers and that the providers respected them, 49% said that their providers included their partners in care, and 28% said their providers were lesbians. In choosing a provider, they were most concerned about a high degree of expertise. Other important factors included a positive attitude toward significant others and the lesbian community, knowledge about lesbian sexuality issues, being a woman, being recommended by other lesbians, and being pro-choice. Community focus groups of lesbian and bisexual women reflected the importance of the client herself deciding whether sexual orientation is recorded in the chart. Participants also wanted to know whether there were any out lesbians on the provider's staff (Saulnier, 2002). Because these findings are contrary to those of earlier studies, further rationale is provided for the current study.

INTERNALIZED HOMOPHOBIA
AND HETEROSEXISM IN THERAPISTS

Whatever the sexual orientation of the practitioner, s/he must learn to deal with her/his own homophobia and heterosexist bias. During the 1970s and 80s, a number of studies began to focus on how heterosexism can impede client change. For example, it was noted that therapists might assume that all presenting problems were created by the client's sexual orientation, with little recognition of the role of societal homophobia or sexism. They may encourage lesbians to move toward heterosexuality or may perceive lesbianism as a symptom of an underlying psychiatric problem. They may be preoccupied with the causes of lesbianism (Riddle & Sang, 1978). Clients' self-denigrating comments about lesbians may go unchallenged. The therapist may collude with the client to "make the best of it", accept certain limitations without question, and treat relationships as if they could never be as valid or healthy as heterosexual ones (Cabaj, 1988). Therapists who are uncomfortable with a lesbian couple's closeness may label it as immature and pathological (McCandlish, 1982). Therapists needing to establish themselves as liberal may divert attention from clients' treatment needs by assuring them repeatedly of their positive views about lesbianism. Others may point out all of the supposed lost opportunities being lesbian carries, emphasize the positive aspects of clients' heterosexual relationships and the negative aspects of their lesbian relationships, and discourage coming out to family and friends (DeCrescenzo, 1984). Finally, Tievsky (1988) noted that the attitude that sexual orientation makes no difference ignores the significance of a rejecting society, and being too accepting may lead to missing important issues and romanticizing the couple's out relationship.

During the 1990s, several articles added significantly to the literature on heterosexist bias. Sanders (1993) noted that heterosexist beliefs are reflected in framing same sex love as a "phase" that the client will "grow out of," assuming that lesbians have no interest (sexual or emotional) in men, and assuming that lesbians are not really sexually interested in one another. McHenry and Johnson (1993) noted that the biases of homophobia and heterosexism are present in all practitioners in varying degrees and, when denied, interfere with empathy and objectivity. Important transference and counter transference issues are ignored, and therapist and client collude with each other to avoid the issues that arouse the most anxiety and pain. "This mutual collusion prevents the knowing and accepting of the real self, and instead fosters the continuation of numerous aspects of self-hate" (p. 143). Therapists may collude with client ambivalence, homophobic statements, and emotional isolation. They may also ignore lesbian co-parents and devalue positive lesbian experiences.

Since 2000, the literature on heterosexist bias has continued to grow. Appleby (2001) has addressed homophobia in the helping professions, and more attention has been given to biphobia (Mohr, Israel, & Sedlacek, 2001). Mohr (2002) developed four models of heterosexual identity for use in understanding their practice with LGB clients. These include compulsory, democratic, politicized, and integrative heterosexuality. Messinger (2006) has noted that all social workers "have internalized to different degrees the homophobia, heterosexism, biphobia, and transphobia that shape current society" (p. 463).

It is well established that lesbian and gay therapists are as susceptible to homophobia and heterosexism as are their clients. McHenry and Johnson (1993) point out that sexual orientation indicates little or nothing about the skill level or self-awareness of the therapist, and some gay and lesbian therapists are more homophobic and thus more harmful to lesbian clients than heterosexual therapists. Certainly, practice with lesbian clients presents a number of challenges to lesbian and gay therapists. Mutual blind spots can lead to collusion to avoid shared areas of conflict, impeding the therapeutic process (Schwartz, 1989). Internalized homophobia can be either under or over-emphasized by the therapist. The lesbian therapist may attribute all problems to societal and internalized homophobia, losing sight of important family of origin and relational issues.

McCandlish (1982) points out that lesbian therapists are particularly prone to idealizing the relationship of lesbian couples, over-investing in the treatment outcome, and over-identifying with the couple. Cadwell (1994) also points to over-identification and anger as counter transference issues of particular relevance to lesbian and gay therapists. Over-identification with the clients' issues can lead to the avoidance of certain feelings or content areas for fear of causing discomfort in the client. According to Fickey and Grimm (1998), "this over-identification can trigger the therapist's own anger concerning feelings of victimization and societal marginalization and result in the therapist's impotence as an agent of change for the client" (p. 83). Sarah Pearlman, a lesbian therapist, has written about her "overwhelming inclinations to rush in, to protect, overprotect, and rescue in order to make their feelings (and my own) disappear" (1996, p. 78).

THE PRESENT STUDY

It has been over ten years since Hartman (1993) called for gaining knowledge from the narratives of experiences of lesbians. Van Voorhis and Wagner (2002) add that ". . . social work journals must increase the number of articles on homosexuality and, moreover, those articles must address practice interventions with the heterosexist conditions that oppress gay and lesbian clients" (p. 353).

The present study explores heterosexism and homophobia in human services in a mid-sized northwest city known to be lesbian-friendly. Particular interest was given to both those service providers who self-identified as providing responsive services to the lesbian community and to the experiences of lesbian families who received services. The authors were interested in exploring the prevalence in practice of the heterosexist bias explicated in the existent literature. This study was approved by the Institutional Review Board of the researchers' University.

METHODOLOGY

Sampling

To explore the potential biases and barriers to services for lesbians and their families, two survey instruments were developed. Practitioner surveys (47) were mailed directly to listings in the gay/lesbian community directory and to those advertising in the local gay/lesbian newspaper. For the sample of service users, a call for research participants was placed in the local newspapers and flyers were distributed throughout the metropolitan area. The local lesbian advocacy group also provided a mailing list. The call was for those who identified as lesbians/lesbian family and who had sought counseling services. Lesbians interested in participating contacted the researchers and were mailed surveys; 311 surveys were sent to interested participants. This approach allowed the researchers to address directly with families any concerns regarding the purpose and scope of the study. The researchers received calls from approximately a half-dozen bisexual identified women for clarification of the parameters of the project, who were screened out of the study, unless they self identified as lesbian, lesbian partnered, and/or raising children with another woman.

Data Collection

The practitioner instrument was a self-administered, twenty-six item survey designed to elicit practitioners' experiences and perspectives regarding their ability to provide appropriate, lesbian sensitive services to clients and their families. The survey included eight demographic questions, fourteen close-ended questions (e.g. "Do you have a lesbian therapist as a supervisor or consultant?") and four qualitative questions (e.g. "Do you believe that lesbians should see only therapists who are 'out' lesbians themselves? Why or why not?").

The family survey was modified after a brief pilot of its effectiveness. The initial family survey was designed and given to 10 lesbian parents who responded to the researchers' study flyers placed in local lesbian-owned coffee shops. The survey was then modified to provide for more qualitative comments for each of the rated responses or to provide additional experiences not captured in the survey questions. The final instrument was a self-administered, 16-question survey designed to elicit participants' experiences and perspectives regarding counseling services for those who identified as lesbians/lesbian families. The survey included 14 close-ended questions (e.g. "Were you self-identified as a lesbian when receiving services?") requesting participants to rate their responses as "Never," "Rarely," "Sometimes," "Frequently" or "Always." These items also included opportunities for comments or clarification by the participant. Additionally, two qualitative questions were included (e.g. "Were there specific experiences that prevented your utilization of services? Please discuss.").

Data Analysis

Qualitative survey data was first divided into small units of content, then sorted into groups containing similar content. Larger conceptual categories were then identified (Lincoln & Guba, 1985). Trustworthiness (validity and reliability) was achieved through the use of peer debriefers and an audit trail of raw data. Close-ended questions were assessed using a five-point Likert scale, ranging from "never" to "always." Demographic and close-ended data were entered into SPSS to obtain frequencies, means, modes, and ranges.

FINDINGS

Practitioner Sample

Of the 47 questionnaires mailed to practitioners, 25 (53%) were returned with usable data. All but one respondent were female; 10 identified as heterosexual, 10 as lesbian, and 5 as bisexual. The average age of therapists was 46, and they ranged in age from 29 to 61. They had an average of 17 years of experience. One had a bachelor's degree, three had doctorates, and the remainder had master's degrees. Ten practitioners were M.S.W.s and 11 had an M.A. or M.S. in a variety of fields. Their theoretical orientations were quite varied, and all but two had been trained in feminist ideology. All but two had received personal psychotherapy, averaging five years. Nine (36%) had a lesbian therapist as a supervisor or consultant.

Practitioner Findings

Practitioners were asked to discuss their therapy with lesbian clients in regard to coming out decisions, self disclosure, homophobic comments made by clients, countertransference issues, and professional bias against lesbians.

When asked if they ever discourage lesbian clients from coming out, only five therapists (20%) stated that they did, if clients were not fully aware of the consequences or if coming out would be dangerous. When asked about their sexual orientation by lesbian clients, only one therapist (a lesbian) said she never disclosed her sexual orientation. Six therapists (one of whom was heterosexual) stated that it depended upon client dynamics, and the overwhelming majority (72%) always disclosed their sexual orientation when asked.

Only one therapist (a heterosexual female) was not sure what she would do to manage homophobic comments made by lesbian clients. The rest stated that they would explore the comment more deeply, create awareness and educate the client, and connect the comment to internalized homophobia and self-esteem issues. Therapists were asked if they experienced differences in establishing therapeutic alliances with more "masculine" or "feminine" appearing clients. Four women (lesbian and bisexual) stated that more masculine appearing lesbians have more problems initially with vulnerability, have stronger protective walls around them, and have an affective presentation that makes it more difficult to form a therapeutic alliance. One therapist (a lesbian) acknowledged significant counter transference problems with lesbians who are more masculine in appearance. Therapists were also asked if they believe lesbians should see only therapists who are "out" lesbians themselves. Only two therapists, both lesbians, answered in the affirmative, stating their belief that early in the coming out process it is important to see someone who can personally relate to your stories. Of those who responded in the negative, two therapists noted that this is important to some lesbians seeking therapy and had actually been important to them in choosing their therapist. Two respondents stated that there are as many homophobic lesbians as homophobic heterosexuals, and four stated that if you are a lesbian therapist, you should be "out."

Finally, therapists were asked if they personally knew of incidences of professional bias against lesbian clients, and almost half (48%) said they did. Several therapists referred to practitioners of reparative therapy, a male therapist who also serves on the board of an anti-gay organization, and a male therapist who told a client she was "possessed by the demon of homosexuality" and needed to have the demon cast out. Other examples included bias by an adoption agency, a child welfare agency, and a court evaluator (psychologist) who made no referrals to appropriate gay-friendly services. There were other stories from clients about heterosexual therapists who don't "get" what it's like not to have heterosexual privilege, and therapists who have disrespected and invalidated them. Some therapists knew of practitioners who make subtle negative comments about "those lesbians", while others equate lesbianism with a history of sex abuse. One therapist knew of a practitioner who assumed that her woman client's extramarital attraction was to a man (she never returned for another session), and one respondent stated that she was in treatment for years with a therapist who never asked about her sexual orientation (she was too uncomfortable to disclose).

Family Sample

A combination of snowball design, newspaper ads, project flyers and the advocacy mailing list resulted in 311 requests for surveys. Ninety-eight surveys with usable data were received. An additional 27 surveys with only partial data were received, and these were not included in the analysis. Thus, 40% of mailed surveys were returned, and 32% of those mailed were usable. The authors are aware that this is a less than desirable response rate, although, according to Grinnell (2001), "it is not uncommon for mail surveys to yield response rates of only 10 to 20 percent" (p. 317). Though specific demographic data were not collected, the researchers hypothesize that these responses reflected a middle/upper middle class economic group. This is because, as noted below, cost, transportation, and child care were not seen as barriers to receiving services. It should be noted that these 98 responses were quite different from the pre-test responses, which reflected more negative interactions with practitioners and/or services. It is possible that the responses of the 98 family members reflected their membership in the advocacy group.

Family Findings

Typical barriers to services for lesbian families such as childcare, transportation, and financial resources were not reported as significant for these participants. However, stigma-related barriers continued to be a challenge. If they had not sought counseling services in the last six months, several reasons were noted:

- "Because they like to put you down for what you are . . . I feel out of place."
- "I often do not disclose" or "I'm very careful who I seek services from and they are not always available."
- "One therapist left to work somewhere else; another therapist left due to health problems . . . I didn't want to start over with someone new again."
- "I don't feel safe to talk openly about my family and the difficulties my son may be facing living in a lesbian household . . . it was just assumed that we were a heterosexual family."

Individuals who were currently receiving counseling services and had identified as lesbian prior to receiving those services believed they had received all the services that they thought they needed. Respondents appeared to have spent time and energy choosing lesbian friendly providers prior to receiving actual services. Many respondents specifically requested gay/lesbian friendly service providers from family and/or friends and spent time contacting these individuals to assess their level of "friendliness" prior to participating in services. The majority (71%) have found providers sensitive to lesbian issues. One respondent noted, "I have an MSW and know how to advocate for myself. I have sought out gay-friendly private therapists. One was a lesbian. The straight women I have seen were feminists and had lots of gay clients."

Of the 28 women (29%) who were dissatisfied with services, 12 responses reflected feelings that their sexual orientation was not respected. This same subgroup also reported that they did not receive all the services that they thought they needed, nor would they recommend their provider to friends or family members. It is interesting to note that these responses were similar to the pre-test responses.

Regarding heterosexual therapists, it was noted that "Most [heterosexual practitioners] just try not to put their foot in their mouth, and straight men, while polite, don't really have a clue." There was some agreement that most providers see things through a heterosexist lens, that professional training is inadequate, and that training can not necessarily help those who have values opposing homosexuality. One respondent commented that she doesn't want to waste her therapy time and money educating straight people about her lifestyle.

A majority of respondents (74%) believed that they had not experienced professional bias. Of the 26% who had, some felt patronized by therapists, wasted time and money trying to help therapists get comfortable, had their request for information ignored and continually ran into client intake forms that listed only options like: married or single, spouse information, etc.

In an effort to identify specific barriers to services, questions were asked such as "Were there other reasons you didn't seek counseling services when you were having life difficulties?" and "Were there specific experiences that prevented your utilization of services?" It appears that this sample of the lesbian population relies on informal support systems to assist them when life difficulties arise rather than seeking services, as reflected in the following comments: "Sometimes counseling isn't always the best option and there are other ways of dealing with life difficulties." "Since childhood I've pretty much had to work things out within myself and talking things over with a close friend at times." "Perhaps growing up in a large family (8th of 10) led to learning to help myself and my parents were spread thin . . . it seemed better not to add to their burdens, just figure things out myself."

Concerns about confidentiality and anonymity also were identified among those who consider this particular metropolitan area a "small lesbian community." As one respondent put it:

> There have occasionally been services I might have used but didn't because of confidentiality concerns, knowing and working with a lot of service providers. The gay community is small . . . limited gay

skilled professionals available, especially in mental health. Sometimes it feels like too many people already know your business.

The ability to form solid connections with a therapist was also identified as a potential barrier. "Thinking about how hard it is to find a good match personality-wise with a counselor . . . the person I went to was nice, but seemed bored and a little distant," or "There was the lesbian counselor who didn't share her orientation with me," or "There was the heterosexual male psychologist who was fixated on healthy male/female relationships. This negatively impacts my trust level."

Another set of barriers that were mentioned by these respondents was related to internal self or relationship barriers. For example, "I don't trust counselors with some of my issues/information. I might seek counseling but safety issues prevent full disclosure or participation" or "I was feeling helpless. Didn't think I had time and money to find a good queer-friendly therapist" or "Partner wouldn't agree or was afraid to reveal specific problems."

Negative experiences with child welfare systems were also identified. "When our children were younger they were mandated into treatment. This was a negative experience and it took several years to be ready to return to therapy" or "When the children had trouble in their teens and got involved with Children's Services, group homes, etc. . . . we were not treated well" or "My opinion of children's services, family counseling through the state child welfare agency or juvenile court systems is that many things could have been handled much better than they were." As Mallon (1998) asserts: "Consumers (gay and lesbian) of social and child welfare services have a long history of facing degrading and humiliating experiences within these systems and harbor great fear and distrust of the system" (p. 25).

Though typical socioeconomic barriers were not reflected in the majority of responses, they did surface occasionally. For instance, one respondent reported:

The far most important barrier is income . . . availability of time . . . access to information and access to transportation. Therapy is marketed to middle/upper income people. It is almost a lifestyle accessory. Most poor people would not consider therapy. There is very limited access. Nor in my opinion are they (or we) welcome when they arrive. Although I have a good income now, I was poor for many years.

In addition to barriers noted, some counselor biases were revealed. Specific examples are as follows:

- "My counselor conveyed a sense that a long term, monogamous lesbian relationship was less valid, and hence, less a real issue for family therapy than a heterosexual marriage."
- "Not long into the initial couple interview, the therapist began to discuss how she believed we 'merged' with each other. I know this is an area some have identified as a 'lesbian problem', but I'm not sure my partner and I have this pattern. Even if we do, her judgment and discussion of it was way too soon and unrelated to what we came to see her about. I felt categorized before she knew us."
- "Services for Children and Families revoked my foster parent license when I came out as a lesbian, despite the positive work I had done." And finally,
- "I came out to a Ph.D. in 1978 and was told I couldn't possibly be gay. Was told I should date more men. I ended up getting married, and it was almost 20 more years before I came out. No therapist asked what my orientation was. All assumed I was straight. Another psychologist I came out to got flustered and advised me to not make 'hasty decisions' regarding divorce. He seemed to consider it a phase."

DISCUSSION

This sample of very experienced therapists came across as quite sensitive to the issues of their lesbian clients, but almost half personally knew of incidences of professional bias against lesbian clients. This continues to be an area of concern, as well as the finding that some therapists report more difficulty in establishing a therapeutic alliance with more masculine appearing lesbians. Of the family members surveyed, only 26% reported stigma (bias) related behaviors on the part of practitioners. This finding is a bit surprising, given the pervasiveness of heterosexism reported in the literature. As discussed previously, however, this is a lesbian-friendly community, and the respondents relied heavily on informal support systems and spent a great deal of time and energy selecting lesbian-friendly providers. It would be interesting to replicate this study with providers and service users in communities that are less openly receptive to gay and lesbian individuals.

For practitioners and agencies in communities that are potentially not as friendly, it is critical to provide environmental cues that establish safety and acceptance. As Mallon's research (1998) revealed:

> Gays and lesbians generally noted the lack of signs indicating that it was safe to be open about their sexual orientation. Just as they looked for cues from staff and peers, they also scanned their environments . . . When they determined that it was not safe, they concealed their identity. (pg. 81)

Although homophobia and heterosexism may be conscious and handled directly within therapy, they can also be hidden and denied (McHenry & Johnson, 1993). As discussed previously, most studies conclude that many therapists are biased and insensitive when working with lesbian, bisexual, and gay clients (Garnets et al., 1991). In the present study, 48% of the providers knew incidents of professional bias against lesbian clients. Family respondents had exerted considerable energy locating lesbian friendly providers prior to accessing services. They believed that most providers saw situations through a heterosexist lens, and 26% had experienced professional bias. This took the form of patronizing behavior, heterosexist intake forms, and provider denial of their stated sexual orientation. Long-term monogamous lesbian relationships were viewed as less valid than heterosexual marriages.

Studies indicate that graduate students often report inadequate education and training in working with lesbian and gay clients, and are unprepared to work effectively with them (Committee on Lesbian, Gay, and Bisexual Concerns Joint Task Force, 2000). Although the Council on Social Work Education requires that programs must include curriculum content on sexual orientation (CSWE, 1992), lesbian and gay subject matter not related to HIV/AIDS constitutes only about one per cent of the social work literature. Most of these articles focus on helping lesbian clients adapt to their heterosexist environments; few address changing heterosexist attitudes, behaviors, or policies (Van Voorhis & Wagner, 2002). Mallon (1998) emphasizes that in working with gay and lesbian youth, written, formal policies help prevent discrimination, harassment and verbal abuse of self-declared gays and lesbians and those perceived to be so. In the present study, practitioners appeared to be dealing appropriately with clients' internalized homophobia, and seemed sensitive to the issues of their lesbian clients. Family respondents, however, viewed professional training as inadequate and doubted that it could modify anti-homosexual values. They saw their personal education of heterosexual providers as a waste of their own time and money.

In reviewing the principles of lesbian-affirmative practice, Appleby and Anastas (1998) point out that the presumption of heterosexuality is the most common therapeutic mistake. It is critical to use language that conveys openness to both a heterosexual and lesbian identity. Family respondents in the present study noted that providers assumed that they were a heterosexual family and stated that one male provider was "fixated on healthy heterosexual relationships." Appleby and Anastas (1998) also state that it is important to assess how the presenting problems are both affected by and separate from the client's sexual orientation. One family respondent in the present study noted that a provider began to discuss a "merging" dynamic between partners in the initial interview which, even if it did exist, was unrelated to the presenting problem. Effective workers also need knowledge about the coming out process, identity development and stigma management strategies, and how to recognize homophobia and heterosexist privilege in themselves and others. Several providers in the present study expressed intolerance for gender nonconformity, reflecting their own heterosexism.

Practitioners may consult a number of books and journals related to lesbian studies. Relevant journals include the Journal of Gay and Lesbian Social Services, Journal of GLBT Family Studies, Journal of Lesbian Studies, and the Journal of Gay and Lesbian Psychotherapy. Additional knowledge in the areas of substance abuse and depression is also helpful. Finally, heterosexual practitioners and social work educators need to embrace advocacy efforts as allies. As Washington and Evans (2000) assert:

> Advocacy in the (educational) institution involves making sure that issues facing LGBT students and staff are acknowledged and addressed. This goal is accomplished by developing and promoting education efforts that raise the awareness level and increase the sensitivity of the heterosexual students,staff and faculty on campus to the barriers experienced by their GLBT counterparts. (pg. 315)

Practitioners wanting to enhance services for lesbians and their families need to work with their professional agencies and organizations to ensure the development of safe, inclusive environments, including forms that do not assume heterosexuality. The overwhelming majority of practitioners in the present study are transparent about their own sexual orientation with clients, and it is clear that this was important to the family respondents. There is a need for more pro-bono and sliding-fee opportunities for lesbian families, and workers should be careful about stereotyping the dynamics of these families.

Reducing internalized homophobia and countering stereotypes about lesbians require an approach that is collaborative and strengths-based. As workers become aware of their own personal biases, it should be noted that one of the most effective means of changing attitudes continues to be personal contact with lesbian, bisexual, and gay people (Eliason, 1995).

Appleby and Anastas (1998) conclude that there is no need to develop a new theory or model of social work practice with lesbians. However, it is clear that no data demonstrate that reparative or conversion therapies are effective; they may, in fact, be harmful (Haldeman, 1994; Tozer & McClanahan, 1999). Rather, an emphasis on support, psycho-education, and empowerment go a long way in reducing internalized homophobia. Workers should be encouraged to obtain supervision and consultation when working with lesbian clients. Although it is a mistake to assume that the most important family ties are biological ones, families are just as important to lesbians as to other clients, and couple and family therapy are often the most appropriate intervention modalities.

Limitations

Although the findings are important in informing practice with lesbians and their families, this study does have some limitations. The 123 participants came from a mid-sized northwest city known to be lesbian friendly. Their responses may not be reflective of other mid-sized communities. In addition, this study utilized convenience sampling. The majority of family participants were identified through a local advocacy group mailing list and practitioners were identified through local lesbian literature and advertisements. These methods of recruitment limit the generalizability of findings. Another complicating factor was that the anonymity of the surveys made it impossible to match the responses of the practitioners with the experiences of the families.

This study does suggest that there is an untapped body of knowledge about what lesbians and their families do to manage life crises if neither covert heterosexism, bias or lack of knowledge hinders access to professionals, nor more overt barriers such as economics, child care or geographical challenges are present. There are undoubtedly larger contextual questions beyond the preparation of lesbian-sensitive practitioners that would explore not only what is working, but who is not being "heard."

REFERENCES

Adams, M., Blumenfeld, W.J., Casteneda, R., Hackman, H.W., Peters, M.L., & Zuniga, X. (2000). *Readings for Diversity and Social Justice: An Anthology on Racism, Antisemitism, Sexism, Heterosexism, Ableism, and Classism.* NY: Routledge.

Appleby, G.A. (2001). Lesbian, gay, bisexual, and transgender people confront heterocentrism, heterosexism, and homophobia. In G. Appleby, E. Colon, & J. Hamilton (Eds.), *Diversity, oppression, and social functioning: Person-in environment assessment and intervention.* Boston: Allyn and Bacon.

Appleby, G.A. & Anastas, J.W. (1998). *Not just a passing phase.* NY: Columbia University Press.

Berkman, C.S. & Zinberg, G. (1997). Homophobia and heterosexism in social workers. *Social Work,* 42(4), 319-332.

Buloff, B., & Osterman, M. (1995). Queer reflections: Mirroring and the lesbian experience of self. In J.M. Glasgold & S. Jasenza (Eds.), *Lesbians and psychoanalysis: Revolutions in theory* (pp.93-106). NY: The Free Press.

Black, B., Oles, T.P. & Moore, L. (1998). The relationship between attitudes: Homophobia and sexism among social work students. *Affilia,* 13, 166-189.

Cabaj, R.P. (1988). Homosexuality and neurosis: Considerations for psychotherapy. *Journal of Homosexuality,* 15, 13-23.

Cabaj, R.P. (2000). Substance abuse, internalized homophobia, and gay men and lesbians: Psychodynamic issues and clinical implications. In J.R. Guss & J. Drescher (Eds.), *Addictions in the gay and lesbian community* (pp. 5-24). New York: Haworth.

Cadwell, S.A. (1994). Over-identification with HIV clients. *Journal of Gay & Lesbian Psychotherapy,* 2(2), 77-99.

Committee on Lesbian, Gay, and Bisexual Concerns Joint Task Force. (2000). Guidelines for psychotherapy with lesbian, gay, and bisexual clients. *American Psychologist,* 55 (12), 1440-1451.

Council on Social Work Education. (1992). Curriculum policy statement for baccalaureate and master's degree programs in social work education. Alexandria, VA: Author.

DeCrescenzo, T.A. (1984). Homophobia: A study of the attitudes of mental health professionals toward homosexuality. *Journal of Social Work and Human Sexuality,* 2, 115-136.

Eliason, M.J. (1995). Accounts of sexual identity formation in heterosexual students. *Sex Roles,* 32, 821-834.

Fickey, J., & Grimm, G. (1998). Boundary issues in gay and lesbian psychotherapy relationships. In C.J. Alexander (Ed.), *Working with gay men and lesbians in private psychotherapy practice* (pp.77-93). NY: The Haworth Press.

Garnets, L., Hancock, K.A., Cochran, S.D., Goodchilds, J., & Peplau, L.A. (1991). Issues in psychotherapy with lesbians and gay men: A survey of psychologists. *American Psychologist*, 46, 964-972.

Gay and Lesbian Medical Association and LGBT health experts (2001). *Healthy People* 2010 *Companion Document for Lesbian, Gay, Bisexual, and Transgender (LGBT) Health*. San Francisco, CA: Gay and Lesbian Medical Association.

Grinnell, R.M. (2001). *Social work research and evaluation: Quantitative and qualitative approaches*. NY: F.E. Peacock.

Gruskin, E.P. (1999). *Treating lesbians and bisexual women: challenges and strategies for health professionals*. London: Sage Publications.

Haldeman, D.C. (1994). The practice and ethics of sexual orientation conversion therapy. *Journal of Consulting and Clinical Psychology*, 62 (2), 221-227.

Harris, M.B., Nightengale, J., & Owen, N. (1995). Health care professionals' experience, knowledge, and attitudes concerning homosexuality. *Journal of Gay Lesbian Social Services,* 2 (2), 91-107.

Hartman, A. (1993). Out of the closet: revolution and backlash [Editorial]. *Social Work*, 38, 245-246, 360.

Herek, G.M. (1996). Heterosexism and homophobia. In R.P. Cabaj & T.S. Stein (Eds.), *Textbook of homosexuality and mental health* (pp.101-113). Washington, D.C.: American Psychiatric Press.

Kite, M.E. (1994). When perceptions meet reality: Individual differences in reactions to lesbians and gay men. In B. Greene & G.M. Herek, (Eds.), *Lesbian and gay psychology* (pp.25-53). London: Sage Publications.

Kitzinger, C. (1996). Heteropatriarchal language: The case against "homophobia". In L. Mohin (Ed.), *An intimacy of equals: Lesbian feminist ethics* (pp. 34-40). NY: Harrington Park Press.

Klamen, D. L., Grossman, L.S., & Kopacz, D.R. (1999). Medical student homophobia. *Journal of Homosexuality*, 37 (1), 53-63.

Lincoln, Y.S. & Guba, E.G. (1985). *Naturalistic Inquiry*. Newbury Park, CA: Sage.

Mallon, G.P. (1998). *We Don't Exactly Get the Welcome Wagon: The Experiences of Gay and Lesbian Adolescents in Child Welfare Systems*. New York: Columbia University Press.

McCandlish, B.M. (1982). Therapeutic issues with lesbian couples. *Journal of Homosexuality*, 7, 71-78.

McHenry, S.S. & Johnson, J.W. (1993). Homophobia in the therapist and gay or lesbian client: Conscious and unconscious collusions in self-hate. *Psychotherapy*, 30(1), 141-151.

Messinger, L. (2006). Toward affirmative practice. In D. Morrow & Messinger (Eds.), *Sexual orientation and gender expression in social work practice: Working with gay, lesbian, bisexual, and transgender people* (pp. 461-470). New York: Columbia University Press.

Mohr, J.J. (2002). Identity and the heterosexual therapist: An identity perspective on sexual orientation dynamics in psychotherapy. *Counseling Psychologist*, 30, 532-566.

Mohr, J.J., Isreal, T., & Sedlacek,, W.E. (2001). Counselor's attitudes regarding bisexuality as predictors of counselor's clinical responses: An analogue study of a female bisexual client. *Journal of Counseling Psychology*, 48, 212-222.

Morgan, K.S. (1997). Why lesbians choose therapy: Presenting problems, attitudes, and political concerns. *Journal of Gay & Lesbian Social Services, 6(3), 57-75.*

Morin, S.F. (1997). Heterosexual bias in psychological research on lesbianism and male homosexuality. *American Psychologist,* 39, 247-251.

Pearlman, S.F. (1996). Lesbian clients/lesbian therapists: Necessary conversations. *Women and Therapy,* 18 (2), 71-80.

Riddle, D.I., & Sang, B. (1978). Psychotherapy with lesbians. *Journal of Social Issues,* 34, 84-100. Sanders, G.L. (1993). The love that dares to speak its name: From secrecy to openness in gay and lesbian affiliations. In E. Imber-Black (Ed.), *Secrets in families and family therapy* (pp.215-242). NY: W.W. Norton & Co.

Saulnier, C.F. (2002). Deciding who to see: Lesbians discuss their preferences in health and mental health care providers. *Social Work,* 47(4), 355-365.

Saulnier, C. F., & Wheeler, E. (2000). Social action research: Influencing providers and recipients of health and mental health care for lesbians. *Affilia,* 15, 409-433.

Schatz, B., & O'Hanlan, K. (1994). *Anti-gay discrimination in medicine: Results of a national survey of lesbian, gay, and bisexual physicians.* San Francisco: American Association of Lesbian and Gay Physicians.

Schwartz, R.D. (1989). When the therapist is gay: Personal and clinical reflections. *Journal of Gay & Lesbian Psychotherapy,* 1(1), 41-51.

Tievsky, D.L. (1988). Homosexual clients and homophobic social workers. *Journal of Independent Social Work,* 2, 51-62.

Tozer, E.E. & McClanahan, M.K. (1999). Treating the purple menace: Ethical considerations of conversion therapy and affirmative alternatives. *Counseling Psychologist,* 27 (5), 722-743.

Van Voorhis, R, & Wagner, M. (2002). Among the missing: Content on lesbian and gay people in social work journals. *Social Work,* 47(4), 345-354.

Van Wormer, K. (2004). *Confronting Oppression, Restoring Justice: From Policy Analysis to Social Action.* Alexandria, VA: Council on Social Work Education.

Weinberg, G. (1972). *Society and the healthy homosexual.* NY: Anchor.

INDEX

Note: Page numbers in *italic* type denote tables